HANDBOOK OF CLINICAL TEACHING

EXERCISES AND GUIDELINES FOR HEALTH PROFESSIONALS WHO TEACH PATIENTS, TRAIN STAFF OR SUPERVISE STUDENTS

NANCY T. WATTS PhD PT

Professor Emerita, MGH Institute of Health Professions, Boston, Massachusetts

Foreword by

Rheba de Tornyay EdD RN FAAN

Professor, Department of Community Health Care Systems, and Dean Emeritus, School of Nursing, University of Washington, Seattle, Washington

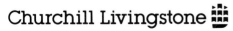

Churchill Livingstone

EDINBURGH LONDON MELBOURNE AND NEW YORK 1990

CHURCHILL LIVINGSTONE
Medical Division of Longman Group UK Limited

Distributed in the United States of America by Churchill Livingstone Inc., 1560 Broadway, New York, N.Y. 10036, and by associated companies, branches and representatives throughout the world.

First published 1990
  Reprinted 1990

ISBN 0-443-03604-7

British Library Cataloguing in Publication Data
Watts, Nancy T.
    Handbook of clinical teaching.
    1. Medicine — For teaching
    I. Title
610'.24372

Library of Congress Cataloging in Publication Data
Watts, Nancy T.
    Handbook of clinical teaching: exercise and
guidelines for health professionals who teach
patients, train staff, or supervise students/
    Nancy T. Watts; foreword by Rheba de Tornyay.
    p.   cm.
    Bibliography: p.
    ISBN 0-443-03604-7
    1. Medicine — Study and teaching.   I. Title.
    [DNLM: 1. Education, Medical — problems.
2. Teaching — methods — problems.
W 18 W352h]
R834.W38   1990
610'.7 — dc19
DNLM/DLC
for Library of Congress   89-980
                                                        CIP

Produced by Longman Singapore Publishers (Pte) Ltd.
Printed in Singapore

FOREWORD

This *Handbook* for teaching in the clinical setting is presented to health professionals at a time of unprecedented challenges. The public is demanding readily available, high quality care at a reasonable cost at the same time as the funding sources for education are becoming increasingly concerned about what is perceived as the high cost of clinical training for all the health professions—allied health, dentistry, medicine, nursing, pharmacy and public health. There is increasing competition among the health professions for providing clinical services and learning experiences. The accelerated rate of the expansion of knowledge and rapid changes in technology requires a lifelong pattern of learning as an important skill and attitude to be developed for every health science student and practitioner. It is with these issues in mind that this volume was conceived and developed as a contribution for all the health disciplines and those who teach in them.

The importance of relevant clinical exposure for students in the health sciences cannot be overstated. But providing essential experiences cannot always be accomplished because of lack of such resources as availability and the costs of providing them. Furthermore, legal restraints and professional boundary disputes may inhibit creativity in providing alternate ways of achieving clinical goals. It becomes incumbent on the faculty member to select and plan practical experiences to achieve clinical goals.

It is during the clinical experiences that students develop their sense of commitment to clients and patients, and apply their knowledge and skills in helping individuals and families toward attaining and promoting health. In the clinical area students master current information and techniques. It should be here that students learn to be active, independent, self-directed learners with the ability to identify, formulate and solve problems; to grasp and use basic concepts and principles; and to gather and assess data rigorously and critically.

Until the publication of this *Handbook* there has been surprisingly little practical advice to help practitioners and health professions faculty to become more effective in the teaching component of the clinical area. To date the educational literature has contained little information about the major teaching problems encountered within the clinical area. These problems are often complex, involving competing demands for the practitioner and teacher for the tasks to be accomplished. Furthermore clinical teaching usually occurs in the public arena open to the scrutiny of others. In all situations the welfare of the patient instead of the student must take precedence, often leading to the needs of the learner becoming lost in the competing priorities for faculty time, energy and interest.

This workbook provides a unique approach for teachers of health professionals, and for health professionals engaged in teaching clients and patients. The clinical examples selected by Dr Watts are designed to assist health professionals in their approach, and most of the examples benefit from a multidisciplinary approach. Throughout this volume faculty are encouraged to work together in partnerships or teams, thus providing the opportunity for the rich exchange of ideas, views and experiences. The commonalities of clinical teaching have been carefully analyzed, and the approach will be applicable to all the health disciplines. Through the use of an interactive style, Dr Watts invites the reader's participation as a learner, thus modeling the effective use of case studies and simulations in providing learning experiences before working with 'real' people in 'real' situations. She stresses clear and attainable learning objectives and, using a consistent format, she models the importance of facilitating learning through the three essential teaching components—acquiring information, providing practice exercises and giving immediate feedback. The needs of the learner are sensitively explored to provide an environment emphasizing positive and achievable goals.

This is a book for those committed to improving their clinical teaching abilities. Health profession educators hold a key responsibility for the preparation of health professionals who manage various important components of patient care. They have the opportunity to help their students gain understanding of the contributions of each health profession and can focus on the ways in which the various members of the health care team should work together for the benefit of those they serve.

R. de T.

PREFACE

This Handbook has hundreds of co-authors. The exercises are the fruits of over 30 years of teaching in continuing education workshops, staff in-service programs and graduate school courses for health professionals who wanted to improve their clinical teaching. The questions, concerns and ideas of these students have guided me each step of the way in my efforts to translate general principles of education into practical guidelines for teaching in the clinical setting.

As I tried to condense my live teaching methods into the written pages of a book I benefited from the advice of a group of experienced teachers from a variety of health professions. I am especially grateful for their comments on large sections of the manuscript to: Kathleen Creedon (dietetics); Suzanne Ames (medical technology); Margaret Alexander, Rheba de Tornyay, Joan Garity and Cheryl Stetler (nursing); Raija Tyni Lenné, Marilyn de Mont and Nancy Matesanz (physical therapy); and Nava el Ad (social work).

The book also has been a family enterprise. The model of teaching it advocates is a legacy from my mother, May Theilgaard Watts, a teacher of rare talents and strong opinions whose many students *never* simply sat and listened. Thoughtful comments on the manuscript from my brother, Tom Watts, let me draw on his skills as an instructional programmer and publisher to improve the exercise format and purge the text of unneeded and unclear words. The illustrations by my sister, Erica Watts, gave life to many ideas I particularly wanted to emphasize by converting them from easily forgotten verbal abstractions to memorable snapshots of the clinical teacher's real world.

My principal co-author for this book has been Barbara Adams, nurse, physical therapist, teacher and friend. Since my work in clinical teaching began she has been an inventive and untiring advisor and test audience. Her clinical experience, common sense and good humor have been essential ingredients throughout my work on this project.

The final phase of work on the book was greatly expedited by the Mina Shaughnessy Scholars Program of the Fund for Improvement of Postsecondary Education. The generous support I received as a Shaughnessy Scholar in 1985 and 1986 gave me the time and motivation I needed for a concentrated effort to pull my teaching materials together and put them into a form that could be shared with others.

Boston, 1990   N.T.W.

TABLE OF CONTENTS

A GUIDE TO THE EXERCISES

activities you could each carry out to help the student take one step towards correcting the problem
- negotiating agreement on the plan in a way that encourages the student to take the initiative
- summarizing the plan in a written contract that covers all the major points in your agreement.

13 *p. 119* **Power sharing—making the little things add up**

Suggest specific things you can do or say as you interact with students and patients to give them a greater sense of control over their own actions, environment and well-being.

Work alone

Follow-up discussion with others helpful

14 *p. 130* **Giving information, directions and advice: the case of the discouraged lecturer**

Plan lectures that:
- focus selectively on the information your listeners need most
- stimulate student thinking and allow immediate use of the information you present
- are timed and staged to avoid interference from student fatigue, boredom and preoccupation with other concerns.

Work alone

Follow-up discussion with others helpful

15 *p. 136* **Showing students what to do: the case of the determined demonstrator**

Plan demonstrations to help students learn complex motor or interaction skills by:
- providing a clear verbal and mental picture of how the task should be performed
- arranging a time and setting for student practice that make it easy to imitate what was demonstrated
- providing timely, individual feedback to each student even when instruction is given to a group.

Work alone

Follow-up discussion with others helpful

16 *p. 145* **Helping students learn on their own: the case of the wide-eyed observer**

Plan observational experiences for your students by:
- analyzing scheduled events at your facility to identify specific things your student could learn from observing selected activities
- describing how you could use pre-sets and advance organizers to focus your student's attention and guide her thinking during the observation even if you can't be with her all the time
- deciding when to use a discovery approach that encourages students to structure and focus their own learning activity.

Work alone

Follow-up discussion with others helpful

17 *p. 152* **Supervising practice of a complex skill: the case of the flustered technician**

Plan how you will supervise a student's early attempts to carry out a skilled task in a realistic work setting by:
- deciding when the student is ready to attempt the performance
- selecting specific verbal and nonverbal techniques you can

Work alone

Follow-up discussion with others helpful

use to coach the student without being threatening or disruptive
- deciding when and how you should intervene if the student makes mistakes.

18   *p. 162*   **Using questions to guide discussions and conferences: the case of the wandering conversation**

Prepare for group discussions and individual conferences with students by:
- deciding how much you want to control the focus of the conversation
- wording some key questions in advance to make them useful for stimulating the specific sort of thinking or valuing you hope the students will learn
- planning how you will respond if the student introduces an important topic.

Work alone

Follow-up discussion with others helpful

19   *p. 174*   **Influencing student attitudes and values: the case of the realistic role model**

Select methods for interacting with students that foster attitudes and values you believe are desirable by:
- identifying attitudes and values you believe will be helpful to the student in the role for which you are helping him prepare
- analyzing your usual style of interacting with students to predict how it might influence their feelings and beliefs
- planning specific ways you could use such methods as role modeling, graded expectations, direct instruction and non-directive discussion to help students examine and develop their attitudes and values.

Work alone

Follow-up discussion with others helpful

20   *p. 184*   **Drafting criteria for rating a clinical skill**

Develop standards for objective evaluation of an observed performance by:
- deciding what specific things you need to see or hear the student do in order to feel his mastery of a particular skill is acceptable
- describing these key behaviors clearly enough so other teachers can interpret them easily and students can use them as a basis for self-assessment.

Best done with a small group

Can be done with a partner

21   *p. 195*   **Rating an observed performance**

Conduct a rater training exercise with a group of clinical teachers to help them:
- improve the validity, reliability and objectivity of their student evaluations
- suggest improvements in the forms they use to record observational ratings.

Must be done with a group

Group size may be varied

22   *p. 204*   **Giving effective feedback**

Apply a set of general guidelines for giving students feedback on their performance during your conferences with them and
evaluate your own style of counseling and coaching students to identify strengths and weaknesses in your present performance.

Must be done in a group of 3 to 5 people

23 *p. 215* **Evaluating student achievement: a self-assessment inventory**

Assess your own performance in the area of student evaluation and
suggest practical ways in which you can help your students learn to assess themselves.

Work alone

Follow-up discussion with colleagues or students helpful

24 *p. 225* **Preparing a list of learning options**

Individualize the instruction you plan for your students by:
- identifying several different ways students could work on a skill they need to learn
- deciding how these activities could be designed to build in differences that match individual variations in the students' preferred learning styles, interests, needs and abilities
- describing the options in terms the students can understand.

Work alone or with a partner or small group

25 *p. 231* **Analyzing your own teaching style**

Evaluate your own current performance as a clinical teacher to:
- identify any differences that exist between the style you now use and the style you feel is ideal for someone with your teaching responsibilities
- identify some of the factors that make you vary your teaching style from time to time.

Work alone on some components and with several other teachers or students on others

26 *p. 241* **Designing an organizational system**

Plan a logical system for organizing a series of related instructional activities by:
- proposing a basis for putting the separate activities into related groups
- proposing a basis for deciding which activities to work on first and how to sequence the others as the student progresses.

Best to do with several other people

Can be done alone

INTRODUCTION

WHY A BOOK ON CLINICAL TEACHING?

Clinical teachers work in an instructional environment that is rich in opportunity but difficult to control, stimulating but often confusing, rewarding but sometimes intimidating. Above all, it is a setting that is full of surprises.

- Important events may be difficult to schedule. Valuable opportunities for learning appear unexpectedly. Plans for teaching may be disrupted by a sudden change in the patient's condition. Many tasks are urgent. Time pressures are great.
- The general theory of classroom and textbook often fails to explain the varied patterns individual cases present.
- Real problems are often complex and their components difficult to tease apart.
- The work assigned to students is often fascinating and obviously worthwhile, but some jobs are inescapably boring, frightening or embarrassing.
- Neither teacher nor student is free to think only of learning, for patient welfare must always come first.

The general literature of education provides a wealth of ideas clinical teachers can use, but because most of this writing has been directed at classroom teachers, the principles presented often need adaptation before they can be applied in the clinical setting. This Handbook is an attempt to help clinical teachers make a sound practical connection between what others have discovered about teaching and their own day to day work with students.

FORMAT OF THE BOOK AND SUGGESTIONS FOR ITS USE

This is a workbook. To use it fully you will need not only to read the ideas it presents, but also to experiment with its suggestions, write in its pages and use the book as a practical tool for examining your own actions as a clinical teacher.

The book is organized around the basic tasks most teaching involves. Each chapter includes four types of material:

- *Information* on concepts, issues, and methods of special importance in this phase of teaching
- *Practice exercises* that ask you to try your hand at applying these general ideas to specific problems
- *Feedback* in the form of comments and questions you can use to evaluate your work on each exercise and
- *Suggested references* that will help you learn more about the topic.

The exercise and feedback sections have special page headings to make them easy to locate, and to emphasize their importance as components of instruction.

The practice exercises are the heart of the book. In addition to guiding your practice of specific teaching skills, in many of the exercises the series of steps you are asked to follow represents a general process you can apply to similar problems in your own teaching.

You and your fellow clinical teachers have a great deal to offer one another. Therefore, many of the exercises use a format that encourages you to work on them with a partner or small group of colleagues. The exercise provides a framework within which you can exchange ideas and give each other helpful criticism and support. If working with others is impractical for you, however, most of the exercises can be done perfectly well alone.

You may want to adapt the examples and case problems used in the exercises to make them more relevant to your own clinical setting, students and professional discipline. Because clinical teachers from different professional backgrounds can benefit from give-and-take about the variety of methods they use, this book uses examples drawn from many different fields. As a result, some of the technical terms may be unfamiliar to you. The clinical procedures mentioned in the exercises may be things clinicians in your field never do—or do quite differently. When this happens, try not to let details of the content that students in the cases are being taught become your main concern. Focus your attention instead on the instructional methods involved. Substitute your own terms and clinical content whenever this will make your work on the exercises easier or more relevant.

TERMINOLOGY

A few additional comments on several terms used frequently in this book may make their interpretation easier.

- *Student.* In most sections of the book this term is used to describe any person who is taught by a health professional. This might be:
  — a patient, family member or other layman to whom you give explanations or instructions
  — another health professional or assistant to whom you provide on-the-job training and supervision, or
  — a student enrolled in a formal professional or technical education program for whom you help arrange and supervise clinical fieldwork, observational experiences or an internship.
- *Clinical teacher* is the term used to describe anyone who works in a health care setting and has some recurring responsibility for students. It is *not* limited to individuals who have been given an official title, such as: Faculty Member, Professor, Certified Teacher, Instructor or Supervisor . . . although it certainly includes such people. Nor is it limited to staff who are employed for the specific purpose of teaching. So far as this book is concerned, you

are a clinical teacher even if your work title is, for example, Staff Nurse or Speech Therapist, and you are employed to give patient services — so long as you also regularly do things to help other people learn.

- *The clinic or clinical setting* refers to any of the wide array of situations in which you may work with patients. This might be anywhere from a hospital emergency room to a clinic office, the solarium of a nursing home or the patient's own kitchen. In many cases, the term also can be applied to such settings as the medical laboratory or the hospital kitchen where patients are rarely present. What all these places have in common is that they are places where real work related to patients takes place, and where teaching is often important but seldom is the 'main event'.
- *He and she* are used at random in relation to both students and teachers. There is little logic in consistently designating either of these varied characters as male or female, and repeated use of phrases such as 'he/she' and 'her or his' is tiresome. Therefore, this handbook tries to vary the pronouns used but to treat them as completely interchangeable.

WHERE TO BEGIN

As you work your way through the Handbook you may want to skip some exercises, or do them in an order different than the one in which they are presented. Choose the sequence that meets your personal needs. However, you will find the exercises most helpful if you begin by orienting yourself to the particular model of teaching and learning on which they are based. This is explained at the start of the first chapter. Please look at that before you plot your progress through the rest of the book.

LOOKING AHEAD

Whether you are an old hand or a beginner at clinical teaching your study of this subject will need to extend far beyond the ideas in this Handbook. These exercises only sample the many skills excellent clinical instruction requires. As you find areas of theory or practice you want to explore more fully, turn to the annotated bibliography at the end of the book. It suggests references that will help you extend your knowledge and think about different approaches than the ones described here.

You will find these bibliographies limited primarily to books, in English, published within the last ten years. Professional journals, monographs, dissertations, older books and publications in other languages all provide a wealth of useful material. They have been omitted from these bibliographies simply because clinical teachers in non-academic settings often find such references difficult to secure.

To supplement the chapter bibliographies, and help you find additional references on your own, an additional listing at the end of the book describes several general references on clinical teaching and a selection of professional journals that regularly include papers on this broad subject.

1 THE EVENTS OF LEARNING AND FUNCTIONS OF TEACHING

THE NATURE OF LEARNING

Consider two familiar definitions of learning.

- Learning is the acquisition of knowledge through instruction
- Learning is a change in behavior that results from experience.

Both seem logical, yet these two definitions lead to very different visions of teaching. The first is a content-centered, teacher-initiated view of learning. Here the emphasis in planning instruction is on choosing the information to be covered and deciding how it can be presented so it will be easy for students to absorb. The functions of the teacher are to select, organize, inform, explain, emphasize and clarify. In this scene the student appears principally as a rather passive receptacle for knowledge presented by the teacher.

By contrast, the second definition concentrates attention on the student, on how his memory, judgment, beliefs and actions can be shaped by events in which he takes an active part. Here the functions of the teacher are to arrange experiences that allow the student to attempt the behaviors he seeks to learn, and to guide the student's actions during this experience to foster desirable changes in performance.

This Handbook combines these two definitions. It regards the purpose of teaching as helping students change; but recognizes that providing information is often one of the things teachers must do to make change possible.

WHAT DOES 'CHANGING STUDENT BEHAVIOR' MEAN?

At first glance this is a disturbing idea. It sounds as if the teacher is expected to manipulate students and force them to do things her way instead of being themselves. This view of teaching is easiest to understand and accept if we realize the behaviors in which we are interested may involve any of an immense variety of different ways of thinking, feeling, or moving; and that the change we seek is usually to improve the student's ability to do these things easily and effectively. The teacher's job may be to help the student to remember important facts more accurately, solve problems more quickly, feel confident rather than afraid, move smoothly instead of clumsily. In each case, however, the focus is on what the student needs to do, not just on information, and the improvement we call learning represents a specific change in his performance.

THE FUNCTIONS OF TEACHING

The purpose of teaching is to influence this process of change. In designing instruction the teacher sets out to plan what she can do to get desirable change in student behavior started, keep it going in the right direction, make the change easy to accomplish and durable once achieved. This means the teacher must think about the process through which the change we call learning comes about. To do this calls for a certain amount of practical courage, for the process of learning is still not fully understood—or at least not fully agreed upon by the many scholars who have studied and written about it over the centuries. Whether visualized philosophically as a growing capacity for perceiving the Good or analyzed experimentally as changes in the DNA molecules of a flatworm, many important features of the learning process are still controversial or mysterious. All this is well worth intensive study by the clinical teacher. However, this practical, introductory handbook will not attempt to summarize or compare the many theories of learning set forth in the literature. The model of learning suggested here as the basis for planning clinical instruction is a very simple one. It emphasizes four general components of the process on which many authors *do* agree, for these provide a useful overall framework for relating teacher activity to student learning.

If we observe what goes on as many different types of learning occur, four ingredients seem to be of particular importance: motivation, information, practice and feedback.

Perhaps the most obvious of these is *motivation*. Certainly students can be taught things in which they have no interest. They can learn without being aware any changes are taking place; and, if the teacher is sufficiently wily, students can even be made to adopt ideas and values they initially attempt to resist. But motivation is a lubricant that makes the machinery of instruction move more easily. At the very least the teacher hopes her students will be willing to attempt learning. If this willingness is absent, the teacher's first task is to try to foster it, to provoke interest, to make the process of learning seem safe and the outcome of learning seem attractive. Here the clinical instructor often enjoys an advantage over the classroom teacher. The outcomes of clinical learning are usually of obvious practical value and the student frequently seeks opportunities to learn voluntarily. The clinical teacher also has many attractive and immediate rewards to distribute when learning is accomplished. 'Your doctor says you can go home as soon as you learn to use these crutches.' 'You'll be much less tired at the end of the day if you learn to lift patients this way.' However, some of the things clinical teachers ask their students to learn are frightening to attempt or confusingly different from previous experience. Motivation is something the clinical teacher cannot afford to take for granted.

The second important event in many attempts to learn is for the student to secure necessary *information*. This information represents the raw material with which the student works during the learned performance. It may take the form of terms to be remembered, rules of procedure to be followed, standards for making judgments, or

principles to be applied in planning. The teacher has three very different responsibilities in helping students secure the information they need. The first is to be selective in deciding exactly what information the student really needs in order to perform acceptably. The second is to decide how the information should be stored for use by the student during the performance. Should it be committed to memory so it will be available simply through recall, or will it be just as satisfactory for the student to rely on reference material when the information is needed? The third responsibility is, of course, to decide how students should acquire the information in the first place. Should we tell them, show them, guide them to written sources, or perhaps arrange opportunities for them to 'discover' the information for themselves through experimentation and experience? Unless the teacher takes all three of these responsibilities seriously, instruction can become bogged down in unnecessary memorization of trivial information. The problem with encouraging students to take time to memorize information of dubious relevance is not that this knowledge will somehow prove harmful. The penalty is simply that this uses precious time that could be spent to far better advantage on one of the other important events of learning.

Availability of information and eagerness to learn are important, but they are not sufficient to create most of the changes in behavior we call learning. Before the student masters the new or altered behavior he also must actively attempt to perform it at least once, and usually several times. To learn to recall the correct spelling of medical terms the student must do more than simply see them on a list or hear them in a lecture. He must actively *practice* retrieving their spelling from memory until this behavior becomes easy and accurate. To learn to feel confident in taking responsibility for important therapeutic procedures the student must not only be told how the procedures are to be done, but must have a chance to actively experience a feeling of success when he carries them out. Calculating medication dosage, formulating a care plan, assisting a patient to turn over in bed, reporting observations during rounds, fabricating a hand splint and all the many other specialized behaviors students learn as part of their clinical education must be practiced before they become part of the student's performance repertoire. Teaching is far more than simply 'telling'. One of the teacher's major responsibilities is to arrange opportunities for the student to practice the behaviors he is trying to learn.

Finally, observation of successful and unsuccessful attempts at learning shows us that even repeated practice does little to systematically change performance unless at least some of these trials are accompanied by *feedback* or reinforcement. This means that as the student attempts the behavior, he needs to perceive some type of consequence and associate it with his action. This may involve reward or punishment, praise or criticism, or may simply consist of clues that tell the learner how closely his actions matched the behavior he was attempting to produce. As with the other basic functions of teaching, the teacher can help the student receive useful feedback in many different ways, but planning for this calls for thinking that goes well beyond a view of teaching as presentation of knowledge.

The process of learning described so briefly here can be summarized in Figure 1.

In the center of the picture is the student, an active participant in a cycle of events that combine to change the way he thinks, feels, and acts. Sometimes these changes are gradual and the cycle of events must be repeated over and over before learning is apparent. Sometimes the changes are abrupt or the path of learning seems to take short-cuts and combine several components of the process in a single step. On the outside is the teacher, helping to set these events in motion and providing the resources and guidance the student needs as learning progresses. The importance of these basic teaching functions may vary. Sometimes what the student may need most is for the teacher to serve as a convenient source of accurate, well-organized information. At other times the teacher's most important contribution may be to give the student courage to attempt something new and difficult, or to ask a question that provokes the student

Figure 1 The process of learning and functions of teaching.

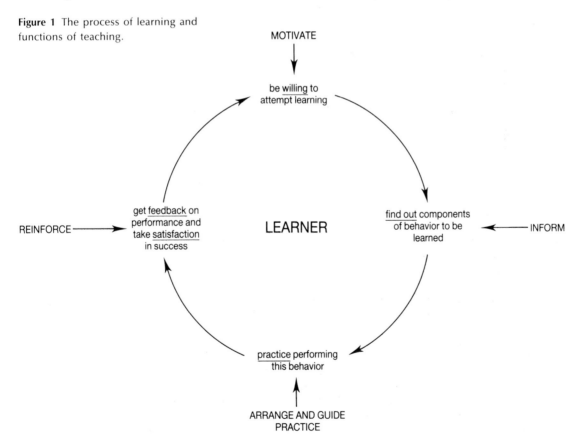

into practicing the type of thinking he is trying to master. Sometimes the instructor simply needs to provide a few basic resources and then get out of the way while the student experiments on his own to find the problems he will solve and the action he prefers.

The guidelines and exercises in this handbook are based on the belief that whatever the teacher's immediate responsibilities may be, the student should be at the center of all instructional planning. Whether the teacher is engaged primarily in helping the student acquire needed information, or in coaching his attempts at action, it is the student he is teaching not the 'subject matter'. Unless the student is changed by instruction, learning has not occurred; and if the student

hasn't learned how can we say the teacher has taught?

This means, of course, that instructional planning must be guided by a clear picture of what we hope to help the student accomplish, of what new skills and values he will have if our teaching succeeds. The teacher does not need to be the one who selects these objectives, but she does need to know what they are before she can help to decide what types of information students really need and what types of practice activities should be most helpful.

Guidelines and practice exercises related to each of the fundamental steps in teaching are presented in the chapters that follow. Because of their special importance in a student-centered

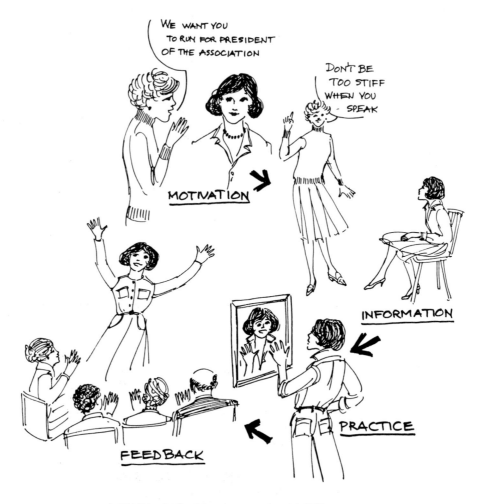

LEARNING TO GIVE A SPEECH

approach to teaching, two functions are singled out for extra attention in this chapter. These are planning for student practice, and planning for reinforcement.

PLANNING FOR STUDENT PRACTICE

The heart of any instructional plan is its design for practice — active practice by the student of the specific behaviors he is trying to learn. The teacher's task is to arrange opportunities for such practice to occur, to nudge the student into action, and to guide the student's performance so it remains relevant. Planning for this is largely a matter of matching verbs, of matching the actions described in the instructional objectives with actions students will attempt during their learning experiences. But in doing this matching the teacher faces an obvious dilemma. The purpose of instruction is to help students become able to do things they cannot do now. How then can the teacher help the student learn to do what he cannot do by having him do that very thing?

When the student is attempting to master a simple new skill or is perfecting a skill he has already acquired at a beginning level, practice can consist primarily of attempts to carry out the full task in its final or correct form. So long as the differences between the desired performance and the student's attempted actions are few in number and easy to see, these remaining problems can often be eliminated simply through repeated trials. But many important clinical skills are too difficult to be performed at an acceptable level of error by a beginning student. Consider, for example, such professional skills as:

- interviewing a patient to take an oral health history
- drawing a venous blood sample
- taking and recording vital signs
- testing the strength of the shoulder muscles
- modifying the components of an enteral feeding.

None of these seem terribly advanced to the experienced clinician, yet before the student can do these things independently in the clinic he must be able to:

- recognize when these actions are called for
- recall the series of steps the procedure involves and the sequence in which they are to be done

- carry out each step with the necessary speed, accuracy, efficiency and confidence;

and, because few clinical skills can be routinely used in an entirely standardized way, the student must also be able to:

- recall how the appropriateness and results of key steps in the procedure should be monitored
- observe and interpret the actual conditions and results of action
- recall recommended ways in which the standard procedure can be modified in response to common variations in conditions or results, and
- carry out each of these modified steps with acceptable speed, accuracy, ease and confidence.

Finally, because basic clinical skills such as these are seldom used in complete isolation, the student eventually must learn to carry out these procedures at the same time as he does several other things; and learn to perform well even under stressful and distracting conditions. To use these skills effectively in the real clinical world the student must be able to:

- reassure an anxious patient as he draws the blood sample
- decide whether to respond to or ignore the page that sounds when he is half-way through an interview
- check the alignment of a skeletal traction set-up and assess the patient's level of general alertness while he records vital signs and makes polite conversation with a visiting relative
- interpret lab data and physical signs while he differentiates among the many formulae available.

Especially when the student is just beginning to learn such complex skills as these, the instructor must invent ways of grading the difficulty of practice activities and of involving the student in performance of the total task by degrees.

SOME METHODS FOR SIMPLIFYING PRACTICE OF A COMPLEX SKILL

1. Guided practice

When actual performance of some steps in the

task is likely to be difficult, the instructor may initially free the student from having to recall what to do and let him concentrate fully on actually carrying out key steps correctly. To do this the instructor provides timely hints, cues, reminders and even direct commands that prompt correct action. This can be done in a variety of ways. For example:

- In the early stages of work on a new manipulative skill the instructor may carry out or demonstrate the procedure at the same time as the student attempts it. The student can then observe and imitate the motions without having to recall what to do next. For example, a nurse might teach a diabetic patient to prepare a syringe for an insulin injection by sitting next to him while they go through the process step-by-step together.
- At a somewhat later stage the instructor may simply need to remind the student of what needs to be accomplished next without showing or telling him how this is to be done. For example, in teaching a student how to calibrate a monitor, the instructor might comment 'OK. You've checked the amplitude setting. Now how would you enter a baseline signal?'
- Or, the prompting may be provided by giving the student a sample of correct work or a set of written instructions to which he can refer if he feels he needs to during the practice activity. For example: 'Here are a couple of correct entries on the cardex and a list of things each entry should include. You may find them helpful as you work on your own recording today.'

2. Mental practice

In other cases actual performance of each of the steps in a task may already be quite easy for the student and mastery of the clinical skill may primarily call for memorization of procedural guidelines or practice of judgments needed to decide when and how to modify the basic procedure. In this event practice may be most efficient if it is focused on the covert remembering and decision-making aspects of performance. Instead of verbally coaching the student through the overt steps of performance, the instructor may ask the student to simply 'think his way through' the task by:

- Mental *rehearsal* of a procedure the student has recently observed or practiced. For example: 'While you're waiting for the staff meeting to begin, use the time to imagine yourself going through the procedure we've just been working on. Try to visualize yourself actually collecting all the materials you need, arranging them in the treatment area, and then actually setting up the equipment so it is ready to use.'
- Mental *anticipation* and planning for events that call for judgmental skills the student needs to practice. The student is often advised to do this at a time when he is relatively free from distractions and not under pressure to respond quickly. For example: 'Before you come on duty tomorrow think about what we should do if this patient's blood gas values haven't improved overnight. How might that show up in his appearance tomorrow, and what will you plan to do if your observations make you think his status is unimproved?'

3. Graduated practice

When the task is too complex or difficult for the student to perform the entire thing initially without significant errors, and separation of physical and mental practice does not seem logical, gradation in difficulty can be achieved through such methods as:

- *Subdividing* the task into several functional sections and allowing the student to practice each section separately before attempting to do all components concurrently or in rapid sequence. In some cases the instructor may do some parts of the task and allow the student to concentrate on one demanding aspect of performance. For example, in teaching a student to ambulate elderly patients using crutches: 'When we walk Mr X this morning, I'll stand next to him to give him support if he loses his balance, and you tell him how he should move the crutches and his feet.'
- Setting *graduated targets* for speed, accuracy or completeness as the student's skill improves. 'This week you will only be assigned to three patients, but by next week I hope we can increase that to five.'

- *Simplifying the conditions* under which the student performs to make them less distracting. For example, providing a quiet place in which the student can practice writing her patient care plans even though staff must usually do this at the busy nurses' station amid interruptions from colleagues, visitors and the telephone.
- Allowing the student to practice a procedure initially in its most *routine* form before trying to incorporate special adaptations that may be needed in practice. For example, letting the student position several cooperative, relaxed patients for an x-ray before assigning him to a patient who is confused, in severe discomfort or unable to move without assistance.

4. Simulated practice

When opportunities for real practice are difficult to schedule, the potential consequences of error serious, or guidance impractical to provide during a real event, initial learning may need to be done through simulated practice. Methods for imitating key components of the real practice situation may vary from the extremely simple to the very elaborate. Examples include:

- Role playing practice with classmates or the instructor taking the part of patients or others with whom the student must interact. For example, this might be used for practice of communication skills such as those needed to cope with an abusive or a very withdrawn patient.
- Practice of physical examination or interviewing skills with actors, lay subjects or former patients who have been specially trained and are employed to portray specific characteristics and to give students feedback on their style and technique.
- Work with computerized or printed patient management simulations or with games that call for the same types of judgments and strategies as those needed for real cases.
- Or simply encouraging students to use their own imagination and experience as a source of hypothetical problems on which they can practice judgmental skills guided by instructor questions such as, 'What do you expect such a patient will be most concerned about when we begin to talk with her about discharge planning?'

To the clinical instructor many of these methods for bringing the level of difficulty of practice activities down to the student's present level of mastery may seem more appropriate for the classroom than for supervised fieldwork. They substitute artificial and contrived activities for the rich authenticity of the real tasks that are so abundant and available in the clinic. These simplified practice activities are also obviously incomplete as a means of bringing student skills up to the level needed for practice mastery. Before instruction is finished students must be weaned from outside guidance and progress to performing complex tasks quickly, flexibly and under the same demanding conditions they will face as graduates.

In designing specific instructional experiences one of the clinical teacher's most difficult jobs is to decide at what level of difficulty practice should be arranged. Will the result of unsimplified practice be confusion and frustration or challenge and growth? Will simplifying the task waste valuable opportunities for clinical learning and deceive the student into believing 'This is all there is to it'? Such questions can only be answered by recognizing that most instructional experiences are part of a continuum, of a series of practice attempts that often begin in the classroom and progress towards the performance we seek through an evolving process of gradual mastery. It does seem wasteful to make careful arrangements for students to do fieldwork in a clinical facility and then to spend much of their time there in role playing, simulated practice or drill on basic steps in a procedure — all things that might be done just as effectively in the classroom. However, it is equally unproductive to thrust students into complex tasks if they are so unprepared for these that much of this time is spent in error and confusion.

STRUCTURING PRACTICE

In addition to selecting and simplifying activities to make sure they are relevant to the objectives and at the appropriate level for the student, the instructor also may need to structure the experience to make it more likely it will actually have the intended focus. Most clinical instructors have had the discouraging experience of arranging for a student to practice an important clinical skill only to find out after the activity has been completed that the student spent the time doing something quite different.

For example, suppose one of your objectives for a student was for her to learn to recognize when patients are showing early signs of clinical depression. To provide an opportunity for her to practice this skill you have arranged to assign her to check the functioning of a piece of complex equipment (e.g. dialysis pump, cardiac monitor, oxygen tent) being used by a patient you feel is depressed. By the time the student's training is complete you want her to look for these signs without being reminded, to judge them accurately, and to do this even when she is in a hurry or preoccupied with some other, technically demanding task. But is she likely to attempt all this today without some initiating stimulus from you? Might she become so absorbed in checking the equipment she forgets to monitor the patient's psychological status? Depending upon your assessment of the student's present level you could structure or direct her activities in any of the following ways:

1. Explicit directions

You can simply tell the student exactly what you want her to pay attention to and do. For instance: 'Before you go in to check the IV on the patient in room 63 I'd like you to think for a minute about what you learned in your psychology classes about signs that indicate a patient is depressed. Then, while you're working with this patient, see whether you think he exhibits any of those signs.'

2. General suggestions

These are much more general instructions, but still provide a reminder that certain types of actions are expected. For example: 'Your patient in room 63 seems a little discouraged today. See what you think when you're with him.'

3. Questions

These too may be either specific and directive or open ended. For instance: 'Did you think Mr Freed in room 63 was depressed when you saw him today?' or 'How was Mr Freed today?'

4. Task requirements or situational stimuli

Often, instead of eliciting the behaviors you want with verbal questions or instructions, you can make use of elements inherent in the activity itself to stimulate practice of the objective. For example, if you know the patient's wife is concerned about his emotional status and that she is articulate and likely to share her concern with others, you might find out when she will be in to visit and try to schedule the student to see the patient at that time. Or, if students are expected to record their patient's progress in daily notes following a problem-oriented format, and you know the format used on this unit directs attention to the patient's psychological status, you may rely on this to structure the student's attention.

For the busy clinical instructor this sort of analytical planning may be impossible for many parts of the student's day. However, when an activity is especially time consuming or difficult to arrange, or an objective especially important, such detailed planning can be very worthwhile.

The following exercises provide practice in applying these suggestions for selecting, simplifying and structuring student practice activities.

MATCHING PRACTICE ACTIVITIES TO OBJECTIVES

This exercise takes only 5–10 minutes to complete. You can do it alone or with a partner or group.

Imagine that you are the primary clinical supervisor for Marcia Hodge, an occupational therapy student. She has just completed the academic portion of her professional education and last week began a six month affiliation at your hospital to gain experience working with physical disabilities. You met with her last week to discuss her interests and to set objectives for her work during the next month. She has expressed particular interest in working with patients who have had upper extremity amputations. Among the objectives you agreed should have high priority during the next several weeks are for Marcia to become able to:

A. perform an initial checkout of a newly fabricated above- or below-elbow artificial arm to make sure the prosthesis fits correctly and that all components are working correctly
B. teach adult patients to use a new upper extremity prosthesis to carry out basic self-care activities.

Here is a list of some activities you could arrange for Marcia this week:

1. Attend surgery to observe an upper extremity amputation scheduled for tomorrow morning.
2. Attend amputee clinic to observe the physician's follow-up examination of a patient who completed upper extremity prosthetic training 6 months ago.
3. Treat a patient who lost his right arm in an industrial accident and who began training in use of his artificial arm last week.
4. Observe while you treat this patient.
5. Meet with you in the staff room to look at several different types of above- and below-elbow prostheses so you can ask Marcia to point out and name the differences in materials and control mechanisms used in these limbs.

TASK A

Review this list of possible activities and rate them in terms of the amount of opportunity each provides for Marcia to practice the skill in objective A.
Make notes of the reasons for your ratings.
Use the following scale to record your opinions:

High	— this activity should allow her to practice all or most of the actions that make up the clinical skill described in the objective
Partial relevance	— this activity could allow the student to practice some parts of this skill, but not the whole thing
Low relevance	— this activity will provide little or no chance for practice of behavior directly related to this particular skill

Then *repeat this rating process for objective B.*

TASK B

Select the activity you rated as providing the greatest opportunity for practice relevant to objective B (teaching the patient to use the prosthesis for self-care). Make a list of any preliminary knowledge and skills you feel Marcia should have before she attempts this activity. These may be things she could have learned in her academic study or things you think she could learn only through practical experience, but all should be prerequisite abilities she needs in order to benefit fully from this assignment. If you feel no specific prerequisites are needed simply write none.

TASK C

Select any one of the other possible activities and write a brief description of at least one thing you, as Marcia's instructor, could ask or tell her to do in order to make her actions during that activity as relevant as possible to objective B (learning to do a prosthetic checkout).

When you have completed all three tasks compare your ideas with those of any colleagues who are doing this exercise with you and with the comments in the following 'feedback' section.

FEEDBACK ON EXERCISE 1

TASK A Match between objectives and activities

Compare your ratings with these:

Activity	Ratings of relevance to	
	Objective A	Objective B
1	low	low
2	partial	partial
3	partial	high
4	partial	partial
5	partial	partial

The closest match between objective and learning activity is obviously between activity 3 and objective B. This activity would permit the student to learn to give prosthetic training by attempting to do this with a real patient. Both the actions of the student and the situation in which the performance takes place are identical for objective and practice activity.

While the fit is not as close for the other activities, several do provide opportunities for the student to practice at least some aspects of either performing a prosthetic checkout or providing prosthetic training. The relevance of activities 2, 4, and 5 to either objective A or B will depend a great deal on how you, as instructor, direct the student's attention before and during these experiences. For example, if activity 5 is limited entirely to asking the student to recall and name components of a prosthesis this is unlikely to have much effect on the student's ability to judge whether a prosthesis fits correctly or to teach a patient how to use the artificial arm to hold a comb or toothbrush. Neither the content of objectives nor practice activity match well. However, by using appropriate questions and directions to structure this activity the teacher can do a great deal to stimulate practice of the cognitive components of the objectives. See Task C in these comments for examples.

Of course there are practical limits to the degree to which it makes sense to try to restructure a largely irrelevant activity. Observing in surgery is probably a good example of such a losing battle. This observation may be a valuable opportunity for practice of some other, still unspecified objectives; but to try to make it a productive experience for learning to check fit or do prosthetic training seems to call for more elaborate and contrived redirection of the student's attention than is worthwhile. Unless the student has already observed a good deal of surgery, this may be a distressing experience. Most of the patient's upper quarter will be obscured, and imagining the prosthesis in place or in use will be difficult. So far as objectives A and B are concerned, activity 1 is a poor choice.

TASK B Identifying prerequisites

In spite of its direct relevance to one of her present learning objectives, activity 3 may not be a good choice for Marcia at this stage in her clinical training. By the time she has completed her 6 month affiliation it does seem realistic to expect her to take independent responsibility for teaching patients to use a new artificial limb, but she may not be ready to attempt this now without special support or preparation. The case description in this exercise gave you almost no information about Marcia's academic preparation related to prosthetics, and told you nothing about her past part-time clinical or work experience. Before you can decide whether to assign her to treat a patient on her own, or begin thinking of ways this activity could be simplified, you need to decide what prerequisite skills the activity requires and to find out whether Marcia now has these.

For example, you might feel that before Marcia assumes full responsibility for this patient's prosthetic training she should be able to:

- establish rapport and interact easily and effectively with cooperative adult patients
- give audible, understandable verbal directions
- recall which self-care activities should be included in early prosthetic training for adult male patients with above-elbow amputations
- recall what the user of the prosthesis must do to move the elbow, and open, close and position the terminal device on the type of limb with which this patient has been fitted.

Inability to do any of these is likely to make Marcia's work with this amputee confusing and upsetting for both her and the patient. You may have thought of other prerequisites that are equally important.

If your observations of Marcia during her first week of clinical work, your conversations with her and your knowledge of her academic program make you feel she has serious weaknesses in any of the prerequisite skills, you should either postpone assigning activity 3 or plan to simplify it using the sorts of methods described earlier.

For example, if her communication and interaction skills seem good, but her knowledge of the training protocol is weak you could:

- rehearse the training procedure with her verbally in advance
- stay with her as she treats the patient to guide her with cues and suggestions if she seems to need help
- model the correct procedure for her yourself by giving the patient initial instructions while she observes and then ask her to continue practicing these activities with the patient
- limit her teaching responsibility to one or two activities you are confident she already knows.

Such modifications as these will allow Marcia to practice some aspects of the total skill at a level of difficulty that presents significant challenge without running the risk of almost certain failure. However, such modifications can only be made if you have given careful thought to the demands the task imposes and have assessed this student's present ability to do what the assignment requires.

Careful analysis of prerequisites and assessment of the individual student's starting level can be equally important as a means of not wasting time on things the student has already mastered. For example, if Marcia has recently written a term paper for one of her university courses in which she did a detailed comparison of the design and materials of different types of upper extremity prostheses, or if she presented a seminar last month in which she demonstrated different limbs to her classmates, she is unlikely to enjoy or benefit from half an hour in the staff room with you reviewing the names of basic components.

TASK C **Providing guidance**

Although activities 2, 4, and 5 do not allow the student to practice doing an initial prosthetic checkout with a real patient, they can be structured to permit practice of many of the recall and judgmental skills such a checkout requires.

For example, before you send Marcia to observe in an amputee clinic you might meet with her to suggest specific things she should attempt to look for or think about while she watches the physician working with the patient. For instance, 'Even though the patient you'll be seeing in clinic today finished his prosthetic training 6 months ago, when the Doctor examines him he will need to check many of the same things that are important in evaluating the fit of a new prosthesis. The patient's stump may have changed and the prosthesis may have gotten worn or broken, so fit and mechanical integrity certainly need to be reassessed. Before you go to clinic it would be a good idea to look over the list of points to be covered in an initial fitting check.You'll find this in the departmental procedure manual. Then while you are observing in clinic I'd like you to try to do three things:

1. See how many of the checkpoints from the initial evaluation list can be covered simply by looking at the patient and his prosthesis as he gets ready for the exam.
2. Then watch what the doctor does to check the fit and test whether the arm is still working correctly. Keep track of how many of the points in the initial evaluation checklist he covers today.
3. Finally, if you think you pick up any problems with the prosthesis, see whether the physician seems concerned about them. If there is time at the end of the examination you can ask the physician whether you were correct in the problems you noticed, or in thinking the fit is still all right if you don't see any problems.'

By giving directive instructions such as these you can help to initiate active practice by the student of the judgmental behaviors in which you and she are most interested. This is often better than simply trusting to luck that such practice will take place.

PLANNING FOR STUDENT PRACTICE

During this exercise imagine you are supervising fieldwork for a student in your own field. The student's present level of performance in one area of skill is described on the attached evaluation sheet. Your job in this exercise is to plan experiences you think will help this student improve her performance in this area.

Please allow about 45 minutes for work on the exercise. It can be done alone, but will be more valuable if you work with a partner or small group.

To complete the exercise please do the following:

TASK A   Arrange to work with at least one partner

Find at least one colleague who will agree to do the exercise with you. If possible, this should be someone who:

- is in the same clinical field as you
- now works or has worked in a similar clinical setting to your own.

If you can arrange to do the exercise with a number of colleagues, form work groups with 3 or 4 members in each group.

TASK B   Agree upon the practical details of your task

Talk with your partners briefly to decide what type of student (professional or technical field) you want Debbie to be, and in what sort of clinical setting you will imagine yourselves to be working.

TASK C   Familiarize yourself with the student

Review the evaluation form attached to this exercise. It records two evaluations of an imaginary student, Debbie Greene. This shows you her current level of skill in only one area: interaction with co-workers. Imagine that Debbie has recently been assigned to your clinical unit and that you have principal responsibility for planning and supervising her clinical work during the next 5 days. You have decided this skill is one that should receive special attention this week. It need not be the only thing you plan to work on with Debbie, but it will be your primary concern during your work on this exercise.

Review Debbie's evaluation to decide what you feel are her current strengths and weaknesses in relation to interaction with co-workers. Symbols used in recording should be interpreted as follows:

S   stands for student self-assessment
CI   stands for clinical instructor's rating
√   indicates this person judged the behavior to be at an acceptable level
N   indicates this behavior was judged not yet acceptable
?   indicates the rater had inadequate opportunity to observe to make a judgment.

Select one specific weakness as the primary focus for a learning experience.

TASK D **Work individually to draft preliminary practice plans**

Use the worksheet attached to this exercise to outline a plan for an experience you feel you could arrange for Debbie that would let her practice the aspect of interaction in which she needs to improve.

This exercise will be most useful if you and your partner(s) begin by doing this independently. Allow yourselves at least 10 minutes to think about what you could do *before* you begin to discuss your ideas with each other. Write down your own ideas on the worksheet as you do this independent planning.

TASK E   **Share your initial activity plan with your partner(s)**

You might do this in any of several ways—by reading each others' worksheets or simply by telling each other what your plan involves. The purpose of this exchange is to encourage you to be specific about your plans and to let you get fresh ideas from one another. Take time to ask questions about anything you don't understand. If you have actually tried out any of these activities with students, tell your partner(s) how they seemed to work.

Once you feel you understand what each member of your group has planned, use the discussion questions on the attached feedback sheet to give each other comments on your plans.

EXERCISE 2

	SKILL 8								Student Name: DEBBIE GREEN

Interacts effectively with co-workers and other health care personnel.

evaluation period

	1	2	3	4	5	6	7	8	Performance criteria: Key indicators for acceptable mastery
S	✓	✓							a. Reacts in a positive manner to questions, suggestions and/or constructive criticism.
CI	✓	✓							
S	✓	✓							b. Demonstrates listening skills (e.g. body language, verbal communication).
CI	N	N							
S	✓	✓							c. Asks relevant and understandable questions.
CI	N	N							
S	✓	✓							d. Communicates information at an appropriate time and place.
CI	?	N							
S	✓	✓							e. Respects the right of those in authority to make decisions by compliance with the decisions.
CI	✓	✓							
S	✓	N							f. Maintains appropriate authority with non-professional staff through respectful, courteous behavior.
CI	?	N							
S	✓	✓							g. Respects time limitations of others by being prepared for discussions, conferences, etc.
CI	✓	✓							
S	✓	N							h. Contributes information to others, being tactful and considerate of others and their views.
CI	N	N							

Does this student now do other things which you feel indicate performance beyond the minimum needed for safe and effective practice or fail to do things which you feel indicate deficiencies in this area? If so, please describe, initial and date.

Eval. 1 – Very shy - has nervous laugh and avoids eye contact when I talk to her. Tries hard to please and is well prepared but lacks confidence. Often too informal when supervising new employees. (BFA, 4/23/90)

Eval. 2 – Seldom initiates conversations with staff, and does not volunteer information in meetings unless questioned directly. Sometimes wastes time getting things done because afraid to ask for help. Seems reluctant to assume authority and give directions or criticize performance of employees she is responsible for supervising. However seems popular and at ease with other students and has a lovely smile (EW 6/8/90)

(Skill rating sheet based on a form developed by the Texas Consortium for Physical Therapy Clinical Education)

LEARNING EXPERIENCE PLANNING WORKSHEET

The principal purpose of this experience is to improve the student's ability in the following specific

area of performance: _____

_____

To allow the student to practice doing this I would ask/tell her to carry out the following tasks: (list specific activities in sequence)

During this activity I would do the following things to provide guidance and supervision:

This would probably take _____ to complete (time)

It should take place in the following setting _____

_____

It would require the following resources (eg. patients, equipment, scheduled staff activities, etc.) ____

_____

Note any other considerations in planning you feel are important on back of page.

EXERCISE 2

FEEDBACK ON EXERCISE 2

Use the following questions to guide your discussion of each other's plans.

1. How closely do the activities planned for the student match the specific areas of behavior in which previous clinical instructors felt she was weak? Do the activities offer her a chance to actively practice whichever of the following you selected for emphasis?

   a. listening skills?
   b. asking relevant questions?
   c. communicating information at an appropriate time and place?
   d. maintaining authority with non-professional staff courteously?
   e. contributing information to others tactfully and considerately?

2. What is there in this activity plan to encourage Debbie to actually practice these particular behaviors? Did the plan call for guiding activity by:

   - direct instructions to the student telling her what to do?
   - suggesting to the student what she needs to accomplish without telling her exactly how to go about doing this?
   - questions?
   - assigning the student responsibilities or putting her in a situation that obviously calls for the behavior you want her to practice?

3. Do any of the plans make use of techniques for simplifying or reducing the level of difficulty of the practice activity to make it more appropriate for Debbie at her present level of mastery?

4. Did any of the plans call for work on prerequisite skills that you felt Debbie needed before she could profit from activities that require her to practice interacting with co-workers? For example, if you suspected her problems arise in part from lack of knowledge of what tasks supportive personnel are supposed to do, you might have planned to teach her this before you asked her to supervise such staff.

You may also have felt Debbie needs some preparatory help in interpreting the performance criteria you and the other clinical instructors are using to judge her interaction skills. She may also need to improve her insight into her own behavior before she will profit from additional practice of interaction. While Debbie and the two clinical instructors who evaluated her earlier agreed on their rating of some aspects of her performance, they disagreed on others. For example, both times she rated herself Debbie checked her listening skills (criterion b) and question-asking skills (c) as satisfactory, while both instructors rated these not yet acceptable. You will find some suggestions for ways in which students can be helped to become more aware of their own behavior included in Chapter 6 of this handbook. Meanwhile, compare ideas with your partner(s) on how you think Debbie's self-assessments might be made more realistic.

PLANNING FOR REINFORCEMENT

Many of the skills taught in the clinic are too complex to be mastered in a single trial. They require repeated practice before all components can be performed with the consistent accuracy, speed and ease needed for independent use. The patient learning to do breast self-examination, the staff nurse learning to monitor patients on a new type of invasive line, and the pharmacist learning to answer physician's questions about drug compatibility, all probably will need to attempt these tasks over and over before their skills become really functional. Usually at the beginning of this learning the student does some parts of the complex task correctly, but omits or makes mistakes in others. One of the teacher's major tasks in designing instruction is to plan when and how repeated practice can be guided so that good points are retained and strengthened while errors are eliminated. Without reinforcement repeated practice will not lead to improved performance.

Unfortunately, repetition and reinforcement are often spoken of as if they were the same thing. A teacher may say: 'This point is really important, so I try to go over it each time I see the patient to reinforce it' or 'Even if I know the students have already had this in class I like to review it myself to reinforce it.' What these statements describe is repetition. They say nothing about how these repetitions will be designed to systematically improve specific aspects of a learned performance.

The simplest way to define reinforcement is as something that occurs in between repetitions to change performance. Reinforcement occurs in the student's experience *after* an attempted performance and makes it *more* likely the *correct* feature(s) of that performance will be repeated next time it is attempted, or *less* likely *errors* will be repeated. Without any type of reinforcement performance may change with repeated practice, but the change will follow a random pattern and it is just as likely to get worse as to improve.

In planning for this component of instruction the teacher must make a number of significant choices. These include:

The focus and type of reinforcement to be used

It may be:
positive — focused on the desirable attributes of the present performance and designed to strengthen them by:

- approval, praise, or recognition ('Good for you!')
- linking some other type of intrinsic or extrinsic reward with the desirable feature of performance ('You're doing so well controlling the position of your ankle I don't think you need to use that splint any more')
- or simply by providing knowledge of results ('That was closer' or a nod of the head).

negative — focused on errors and omissions in performance and designed to reduce the likelihood these will be repeated in subsequent attempts by responding to them with:

- disapproval, rebuke or reprimand ('Come on, you can do better than that!')
- withdrawal of rewards or administration of some type of punishment linked with the specific error ('I can't recommend you for a senior position until your care plans are more complete')
- or with simple, impersonal information pointing out errors in performance ('You're not bending your right knee quite far enough').

The source of reinforcement

Regardless of its focus and type reinforcement may come from:

- the teacher
- classmates, colleagues, family or others
- the student himself if he compares his own performance with a procedural standard he has been given or invented for himself, or when he sees the practical consequences of his own actions.

While reinforcement from other sources is not as easy for the teacher to control as that which he provides himself, the teacher can help in many ways to elicit and encourage such expanded feedback. By allowing time for staff to compare ideas and approaches, encouraging family members to notice modest improvements in a patient's performance, and arranging for students to practice a new task initially under conditions that make success likely, the teacher can greatly increase the variety and potency of feedback these learners receive.

Timing

Both the frequency and immediacy with which reinforcement follows attempts at performance must be considered in designing instruction. The reinforcement may be:

- *continuous*, that is, given after each attempt
- *intermittent*, given after only some attempts
  - at regular intervals (e.g. at the end of each practice period) or
  - on an irregular schedule the student cannot anticipate.

Scope

The number and variety of specific components of performance on which the student receives reinforcement at one time may also vary from

- *isolated* reinforcement of one factor at a time to
- *concurrent* reinforcement of a number of different factors in combination or in rapid sequence ('Overall, you're doing a lot better with your new diet' or 'Your progress notes were much more complete this week, and your presentation at rounds was well prepared, but you're still falling behind on your schedule').

The research literature in education and psychology is filled with valuable studies of the effects of different patterns of reinforcement. Despite this, considerable uncertainty remains about which approach is best in many practical situations. What is clear is that the effectiveness of any approach is likely to depend on the type of task being practiced, the conditions under which this practice occurs, the present level of mastery achieved by the student, and a variety of personal student characteristics. All this makes nonsense of hard and fast specific rules for giving reinforcement. However, some flexible principles can be suggested. Some of the more general guidelines that can be derived from studies of reinforcement, and a few of the dilemmas application of these guidelines may produce, are as follows:

1. While both positive and negative reinforcement can be highly effective in shaping performance towards mastery, negative reinforcement may also promote unwanted secondary learning or side-effects. This is especially likely to occur when the negative response involves personalized disapproval, repeated feelings of failure or withdrawal of highly valued rewards. Although the student may improve quickly in the specific skill being taught, he may also learn to dislike and avoid tasks that call for this skill, learn to fear situations in which his performance can be judged by others, or learn to mistrust his own ability to master new skills. Moreover, learned anticipation of negative reinforcement may create such a high level of anxiety that the student is distracted from the task at hand and even rich opportunities for practice do little to improve performance. The following techniques may help to reduce these problems:

- Focus reinforcement primarily on what the student does right—even if these components of the performance are still far from perfect. Use negative reinforcement primarily to alert the student to errors that are potentially dangerous and when the consequences of error will be obvious and highly frustrating to the student. In general try to eliminate errors by letting them wither through lack of attention and by strengthening correct actions to replace them.
- Recognize that some errors may be receiving significant positive reinforcement from sources outside of your view or control. When an error seems particularly difficult to correct, suspect it may be supported by some type of conscious or unconscious secondary gain for the student. Similarly, when positive reinforcement seems ineffective in strengthening desired features of performance, you should suspect that what you see as correct action may result in some type of punishment from another source. The important thing is to avoid tunnel vision in thinking about the reinforcement your students receive. Even if you are not able to control these outside gains and losses, you can at least recognize when you need to make your own positive reinforcement more competitive in order for it to influence performance.

- Depersonalize negative feedback. Direct criticism at the specific errors in performance rather than at the person who commits the errors. Avoid timing or phrasing such feedback so that it is embarrassing. Help students feel it is 'safe' to let you see their uncertainties and errors while they are learning. Reduce the student's feelings of powerlessness by helping them learn to judge their own performance and by suggesting constructive changes rather than just pointing out flaws. All this may help to diminish the undesirable side-effects of negative reinforcement.
- Set realistic short-term goals for improvement and make sure the student knows what they are. Try to provide opportunities for the students to see evidence of their own progress, even though their overall mastery of the complex skill is still far from complete.

2. Reinforcement is most potent when it is received soon after an attempted performance and can be clearly linked with specific correct or incorrect features of that performance. Delayed reinforcement may have little impact or be associated by the student with some aspect of performance different from the one it was intended to strengthen or eliminate. However, when the student is trying to assess his own performance under realistic clinical conditions, such instant, unambiguous feedback simply may not be available. If the teacher compensates for this by continuing to provide effective feedback himself, the short-term effect may be fine, but the longer-term result may be continued dependency on the instructor. Particularly in the later stages of learning when the student is ready to be weaned from artificial sources of reinforcement, plan for some practice that is accompanied by uncertainty and delayed knowledge of results. Opportunities for students to learn to 'muddle through' on their own may be essential for building independence.

3. Although the most rapid improvements in performance are often produced by continuous reinforcement, the learning created by this strategy also tends to deteriorate quickly once reinforcement is withdrawn. Mastery is most likely to endure when it is acquired through practice in which only some of the correct attempts are reinforced and in which reinforcement occurs on an unpredictable schedule. A planned progression from continuous reinforcement early in learning to infrequent and irregular feedback as learning advances promotes both early success and lasting mastery.

4. Reinforcement is a tool with multiple uses. Because much of the most widely reported research on its use has been done with laboratory animals and with children and adults with learning disorders and behavior problems, reinforcement is sometimes characterized as a soulless technique for imposing the instructor's will on helpless subjects. Reinforcement is rejected by some educators as demeaning, manipulative, or useful only for development of low-level, stereotyped patterns of performance. Certainly reinforcement could be used in these unappetizing ways. However it is also a powerful tool for encouraging individual experimentation, teaching students to analyze and criticize established doctrine, and for fostering the student's attempts to explore personal values and set personal priorities. Reinforcement can be used to 'teach students to behave like programmed rats'. It can also be used to teach students to think and speak for themselves. It all depends on which types of behavior the teacher and the rest of the student's environment reinforce. As in designing the practice components of instruction, planning for reinforcement begins with a clear identification of the behavioral outcomes sought, and should be guided by a logical strategy for action.

The following exercise provides practice in choosing and applying such a reinforcement strategy.

PLANNING A REINFORCEMENT STRATEGY

This exercise will allow you to practice making practical decisions about:

- which specific behaviors to reinforce
- what types of reinforcement to use
- and when and by whom reinforcement should be provided

by working with a brief case problem in patient and family teaching. You may do this alone or compare results with a partner or group. Allow 20 to 30 minutes to do Tasks A–H on your own before you discuss them with others.

TASK A

Begin by *reading the attached case* and the 'script' it includes for one part of a patient-family teaching session. In this initial reading simply try to get an overall picture of the people and activities the case involves.

TASK B

Then go back and take a much closer look at the list of objectives in the background section of the case. In each of these objectives *underline the verb* and not more than one or two other key words that describe the actions Maureen wants to help Mrs Lake learn to perform. Reinforcement needs to follow Mrs Lake's successful and unsuccessful attempts to do these specific things, so you need to be sure you know what they are. Think about how Maureen can recognize attempts at these actions when they occur.

TASK C

Next, on the script itself, *circle at least one phrase* that describes something Mrs Lake did or said that you think *represents an attempt at the type of action you underlined* in objective 1. Write a 1 over each section of the script you circle for that objective. Then *do the same thing for each of the other objectives.*

TASK D

Now *rate* each of the actions you circled.

- put a + sign next to the number of the objective if you feel the action is a positive indicator of learning, an action you hope will be repeated in the future. These may not describe the ideal performance: so long as the action represents some aspect of mastery that should be encouraged in the future mark it +.
- put a − sign next to the number of the objective over any phrase you feel describes an error in

performance or failure to do the sort of thing that is called for by the objective. Use this to designate actions you hope to discourage or eliminate in future performance.

TASK E

Select at least one of the actions you rated as +.
Imagine that you are the instructor, Maureen. Think about what you as the instructor could do or say to give positive reinforcement to this action.

Write what you would do or say in a small balloon over the point in the script at which you would do this. Draw an arrow from the balloon to the script to show exactly where your action fits. If you would prefer to substitute something for what Maureen did or said, cross out the words describing her actions and put the balloon in over that section of the script.

For example:

You're right Mr Lake! She was.

Maureen: ~~Do you want to try that~~?

Do this with as many + actions as you wish.

TASK F

Now select at least one action you marked as – for an objective. Think of one way you could give negative reinforcement to this action to make it less likely to be repeated in future performances by Mrs Lake.

Write this action into the script with a balloon.

Do this with as many – actions as you wish.

TASK G

So far your planning has been entirely related to what the instructor might do or say to reinforce Mrs Lake's behavior. Now try to think of at least one point at which Maureen might have helped Mrs Lake get either positive or negative reinforcement from some *other* source.

Write a note to yourself describing who or what could provide this alternative reinforcement, and explaining what Maureen could do to help ensure this really happens. Note the point in the script at which you think Maureen could do this.

TASK H

Finally, think about the overall strategy you would prefer to use for reinforcement if you were responsible for instructing Mrs Lake during the next day or two.

- What balance would you try to achieve between positive and negative reinforcement?
- Would you usually give reinforcement as soon as a significant correct or incorrect component of performance appears, wait to do this until Mrs Lake has finished a complete phase of the task and there is a natural pause, or wait to sum things up at the end of the full session?
- How much would you take responsibility for providing reinforcement yourself and how much

would you try to encourage feedback from Mrs Lake's husband or try to teach Mrs Lake to assume herself?
- Would you try to reinforce actions related to all four objectives in a single session or focus on just one or two?
- Why do you prefer this reinforcement strategy?
- Do you expect your preferences would change as the time for Mrs Lake to be discharged comes close?

THE CASE OF THE UNCERTAIN WIFE

Characters: **Maureen Arnold**—a staff nurse or therapist on the neurology unit of a general hospital

Arthur Lake—a 67-year-old, retired insurance agent who has been an in-patient on the unit since he suffered a stroke 10 days ago. He is now medically stable and alert, but still has a partial left hemiplegia.

Ruth Lake—his 62-year-old wife, a former public school music teacher who continues to give private piano lessons to a few children in her home.

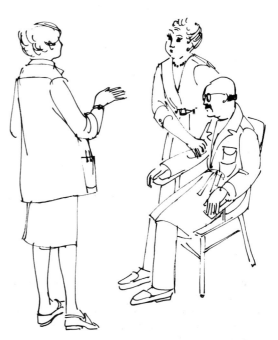

Background: In preparation for Mr Lake's discharge to his home Maureen has been teaching his wife how to assist him in basic transfer and self-care activities. Maureen has now worked with Mrs Lake twice, and feels she has made progress in some areas. However, Maureen is concerned because Mrs Lake still seems very anxious about caring adequately for her husband when he comes home.

EXERCISE 3

OBJECTIVES

By the time her husband is discharged, Maureen wants Mrs Lake to be able to:

1. give her husband clear, step-by-step verbal reminders of how to do the following activities with only slight physical support from her: get in and out of bed, on and off the toilet, in and out of an armchair, and to walk at least 3 steps from bed to chair

2. position herself so she can safely support her husband if he starts to lose his balance during these activities

3. encourage her husband to carry out these activities at home even if they are frustrating for him at first

4. and feel confident in her ability to do these things effectively when her husband comes home.

Scene: Mr Lake's semi-private hospital room. He is seated in an armchair next to his bed, dressed in pyjamas, robe, and slippers. His wife is in a chair next to him, opening his mail and reading it to him. Maureen enters.

Maureen   *Good morning Mrs Lake. How are you today?*

Ruth Lake   *Oh hello. I'm fine. Just fine thank you.* (Smiles at Maureen.)

Maureen   *Hi Mr Lake.* (Turns to Mrs Lake.) *He ate an enormous breakfast this morning so he ought to be full of energy for our practice.*

Ruth Lake   *Yes. He keeps telling me he wishes I'd learn to make those good bran muffins they have here for breakfast.*

Maureen   *OK Mrs Lake. Let's start by going over some of the things we worked on yesterday. Suppose we start with helping Mr Lake get out of an armchair like the one he's sitting in now.* (Pauses briefly.) *Can you show me how you would do that?* (Looks expectantly at Mrs Lake and waits.)

Ruth Lake   *Oh. Let's see. . .* (Pauses and frowns uncertainly.) *Um, I guess I stand here don't I?* (Moves to stand next to her husband's right arm, pauses and looks at Maureen, then turns back to her husband.) *Arthur, I think you're supposed to pull your feet in under you.* (Arthur does this.) *Now, hold onto the arm of the chair with your good hand.* (Looks over at Maureen again.) *All right honey, come on, try to push yourself up.* (Mr Lake pushes and Mrs Lake pulls but he does not succeed in standing.)

Mr Lake   (Grunts.) *Wait a minute.*

Ruth Lake   *Oh dear. That wasn't very good!* (Looks apologetically at Maureen.)

Maureen   (Has noticed Mr Lake is leaning quite far back in the chair and Mrs Lake is standing on the wrong side so her efforts to help interfere with his attempts to push with his good arm.) *Let's try again, but before you start, try to remember how you did this yesterday. Was anything different?*

Arthur Lake   *I think she was on my other side.*

Maureen   *Do you want to try that?*

Ruth Lake   *Oh yes, I guess I got it all turned around.* (Goes to Mr Lake's left side.) *I hope this works. Come on Arthur!* (Pulls on his weak arm.)

Arthur Lake   (Still leaning back too far to get his weight under him easily, pushes hard, fails to get up the first time, but then pushes harder and manages to stand.) *Whew! Made it!*

Maureen   *Now let's see if you can steady him so he doesn't fall while he takes one step over to the bed. Remember, you don't really have to hold him up, just help him balance. Do you remember where to put your hand?*

Ruth Lake   *I think I put it here.* (Reaches around her husband's back to support him at the waist.)

Maureen   *Now Mr Lake, let's move over to your bed. You can reach out for it with your hand.*

. . .and so the lesson continues for another twenty minutes.

EXERCISE 3

FEEDBACK ON EXERCISE 3

TASK B

Key words in the objectives that describe the *actions* Mrs Lake needs to practice are:

1. give verbal reminders
2. position herself
3. encourage her husband
4. feel confident.

   You may have underlined additional qualifying terms as well, but they are not as important in determining the main intent of the objectives. In the first two objectives the key phrases describe specific, *overt* actions—things Maureen can see or hear Mrs Lake do. This makes it easy for Maureen to tell when a successful or unsuccessful attempt has occurred and might be reinforced. While the third objective does not describe a specific overt action, most of the ways in which one person can encourage another to do something are quite easy to see or hear. However, the key action for objective 4 is *covert*. This doesn't necessarily mean that Mrs Lake is trying to hide her feelings from Maureen, it simply means those feelings cannot be observed directly. To judge how confident Mrs Lake feels as she goes through specific steps in the procedure Maureen will need to look for things she does, or fails to do, that serve as indicators of her feelings. In this case the task is not too difficult. For example, if Mrs Lake responds quickly and definitely to Maureen's questions and directions, if she does some things without being told, or if she occasionally disagrees with Maureen's recommendations or makes suggestions of her own, Maureen is likely to infer that Mrs Lake feels confident. On the other hand, if Mrs Lake frequently asks whether her actions are correct, responds to Maureen's questions and directions hesitantly, or reacts to corrections submissively and with apologetic words or facial expressions Maureen will probably interpret these observable actions as evidence of continued lack of confidence.

TASKS C & D

Some of the most obvious positive and negative things Mrs Lake did are marked on the following section of the script.

Ruth Lake   *Oh. Let's see. . .* (Pauses and frowns uncertainly.) *Um, I guess I stand here don't I?* ⁻4
(Moves to stand next to her husband's right arm, pauses and looks at Maureen, then turns back to her husband.) *Arthur, I think you're supposed to pull your feet in under you.* ⁻2 ⁻4 ⁻4,⁻3 +1
(Arthur does this.) *Now, hold onto the arm of the chair with your good hand.* (Looks over at Maureen again.) *All right honey, come on, try to push yourself up.* (Mr Lake pushes and Mrs Lake pulls but he does not succeed in standing.) +1 +1,+3

Mr Lake   (Grunts and says.) *Wait a minute.*

Ruth Lake   *Oh dear. That wasn't very good!* (Looks apologetically at Maureen.) ⁻3,⁻4

Maureen	(Has noticed Mr Lake is leaning quite far back in the chair and Mrs Lake is standing on the wrong side so her efforts to help interfere with his attempts to push with his good arm.) *Let's try again, but before you start try to remember how you did this yesterday. Was anything different?*
Arthur Lake	*I think she was on my other side.*
Maureen	*Do you want to try that?*
Ruth Lake	*Oh yes, I guess* (I got it all turned around.) [−4] ((Goes to Mr Lake's left side.)) [+2] (I hope this works.) [−3/−4] (Come on Arthur!) [+3] (Pulls on his weak arm.)
Arthur Lake	(Still leaning back too far to get his weight under him easily, pushes hard, fails to get up the first time, but then pushes harder and manages to stand.) *Whew! Made it!*
Maureen	*Now let's see if you can steady him so he doesn't fall while he takes one step over to the bed. Remember, you don't really have to hold him up, just help him balance. Do you remember where to put your hand?*
Ruth Lake	(I think) [−4] I (put it here. (Reaches around her husband's back to support him at the waist.)) [+2]
Maureen	*Now Mr Lake, let's move over to your bed. You can reach out for it with your right hand.*

You may have marked your script somewhat differently, especially for actions that are logically related to more than one of the four objectives. For example, in the first line you may have interpreted Mrs Lake's frown and uncertain 'Oh, Let's see. . .' as actions that showed she couldn't remember how to position herself and rated it −2; or as reflecting inability to remember what instruction to give and rated it −1.

Your ratings might also have been different if you are unsure how Mrs Lake should perform this particular activity, or if you disagree with Maureen about such things as where Mrs Lake should stand. So far as this exercise is concerned such differences don't matter. The important thing is that in reviewing the script you tried to compare the actions in the objectives and those in Mrs Lake's real performance.

Although the instructions for this exercise asked you to mark the things Mrs Lake actually did that represent attempts to perform the actions Maureen wants her to learn, you may also have circled some points in the script at which her failure to act was just as significant. For example:

- in her initial instructions to her husband Mrs Lake forgot to tell him to lean forward in the chair before he tried to push up. You might have rated this as −1.
- after her husband's first unsuccessful attempt to stand Mrs Lake made no attempt to encourage or reassure him. You might have rated this −3.
- When Maureen asked Mrs Lake if she had done anything different the day before, Mrs Lake took no apparent notice of the fact that her husband volunteered a correct answer. This means she passed up a good chance to endorse and encourage his initiative. You might have rated this failure to act −3.

The script includes a number of other points at which Mrs Lake's failure to give an instruction or to encourage her husband are significant.

TASKS E through H

Maureen's strategy for reinforcing Mrs Lake's successful attempts at action seems very non-directive. At least so far as her actions are outlined in the script Maureen provides no verbal or non-verbal approval or disapproval, no feedback or corrections on Mrs Lake's actions, and no punishment or reward associated with her performance. Instead of providing reinforcement herself Maureen appears to be trying to get Mrs Lake to assess her own performance so she can provide her own feedback. Even this is done very gently by simply asking Mrs Lake to stop and think whether what she is doing today is at all different from what she did yesterday. In deciding how and when you might give additional positive and negative reinforcement (Tasks E and F) you have many different options. In deciding how to respond to specific things Mrs Lake did or failed to do you will be most likely to choose wisely if you have given some thought in advance to the general strategy that seems best for this particular student at this point in her training. For example, during her first attempt to give her husband instructions at the point when Mrs Lake looks at Maureen after telling her husband to pull his feet in and put his good hand on the arm of the chair:

- If you feel that at this stage in her training Mrs Lake would benefit most from frequent, immediate, positive feedback from the instructor you might have inserted a comment from Maureen, such as: *'That's right Mrs Lake. It's important for him to do both those things.'* Or, you might have relied more heavily on non-verbal feedback, and simply inserted: *'Maureen nods and smiles encouragingly.'*
- On the other hand, if your strategy was to help Mrs Lake avoid making mistakes that could be frustrating for both her and her husband, you might have concentrated on pointing out any key errors. In that case your additional reinforcement might have been something such as: *'**Maureen** — You've forgotten to tell him to lean forward before he tries to push up. That's going to make it very difficult for him.'* Or you might have preferred a less critical comment, such as: *'**Maureen** — That's good so far, but you also need to remind him to lean forward in the chair before he pushes up.'*
- If you agreed with Maureen's emphasis on encouraging Mrs Lake to assess her own performance, when Mrs Lake looks at Maureen you might want to have Maureen avoid showing any reaction. Instead, you might suggest Maureen say: *'Stop a minute and look at your husband's position now. Does he look as if he's in a good position to get up?'* Of course such a question implies that something has been overlooked, but it does give Mrs Lake responsibility for trying to decide what.
- Another strategy might be to make greater use of Mr Lake as a source of reinforcement. For example, you might have inserted: *'**Maureen** — Mr Lake, what do you think? Do you feel as if you're in a good position to start getting up?'* If you decide to take this approach, you would also probably want to make some changes earlier in the script. Apart from her brief 'Hi Mr Lake' soon after she entered his room, Maureen has made no attempt to interact with the patient. In fact, until he volunteers an answer to a question several minutes after the treatment session has begun, we might suspect Mr Lake is seriously aphasic or too confused to communicate. Maureen's comment to his wife on his good appetite, although cheerful, sounds more like something one might say about a very small child than a comment to be made over the head of a retired businessman. If Maureen wants to involve the patient as a partner in this activity, she will need to make a variety of changes in her style.
- In addition to making such decisions about the type and sources of reinforcement to be emphasized, you need to make some practical choices of timing. For instance, instead of inserting additional reinforcement immediately following each positive or negative action, you might plan to reinforce selectively and respond only to those actions you feel it is important to influence first. Or you may decide not to interrupt the flow of Mrs Lake's action with comments and wait until there is a natural pause when you can give slightly delayed feedback on several points at one time.

In this case some types of strategy are obviously inappropriate. For example, there seems little point in attempting to increase Mrs Lake's self-confidence by negatively reinforcing the many things she does that reflect uncertainty. If Maureen tells Mrs Lake to '_stop looking over to see what I think all the time,_' this may discourage Mrs Lake from revealing how she feels. However, she may feel less sure of her own skills than ever. A more promising approach would be to ignore her questioning looks, hesitation and self-critical remarks and concentrate instead on giving positive reinforcement to actions that reflect some feeling of confidence.

Other choices may be more difficult. A logical strategy is especially difficult to plan when each of the various approaches we might choose seems to offer advantages in terms of some objectives and disadvantages for others. For instance, because Mrs Lake has only recently begun learning to help her husband with functional activities, and obviously is still very unsure of herself, it is tempting to try to reduce her anxiety by giving her lots of immediate, strong, positive feedback. This may help her learn to position herself and give clear instructions quickly. However, it may also increase her dependence on Maureen. Will this approach make Mrs Lake unable to see flaws in her own performance? Will her mastery of the techniques deteriorate rapidly once Maureen is not available to bolster the performance with praise? These are not easy questions to answer, but they do at least need to be considered in deciding whether reinforcement should be frequent and positive early in training and then progress towards greater reliance on self-assessment or whether it would be best to emphasize self-assessment from the very start.

Regardless of the approach to reinforcement Maureen uses initially, by the time her husband is discharged Mrs Lake needs to be able to perform well without instructor feedback. When she is on her own at home Mrs Lake must be able to detect any mistakes that creep into her performance and she must be persistent in working with her husband even when no one else is there to praise her efforts. Fortunately Mrs Lake is herself an experienced teacher and used to evaluating the motor performance of others, but unless Maureen can wean Mrs Lake from reliance on outside feedback, problems in compliance with the regimen she has learned seem almost certain.

As a clinical teacher you will need to achieve this same sort of independence. Your repeated practice of giving reinforcement will lead to steady improvement in this important skill only if you use feedback from others wisely and learn to think critically about your own performance. To do this, pause from time to time to think about the specific ways in which you are giving reinforcement to an individual student. Consider the following questions:

- How would you characterize the pattern of reinforcement you are using? What type, sources and timing of reinforcement does it employ?
- Is the pattern logical? Can you explain why this particular pattern is preferable at this point for this student? Are your actions really consistent with this rationale?
- Do you have a plan for helping your students become independent of you by teaching them to evaluate their own performance?

2 DECIDING WHAT YOUR STUDENTS WANT AND NEED TO LEARN

CONCERNS AND CONSTRAINTS

Clearly defined objectives are essential tools for planning instruction. They are the basis for deciding:

- what information to present
- what practice activities to arrange
- what student actions to reinforce

and objectives serve as a standard by which teachers and students can judge the success of their efforts. Deciding exactly what students need to learn is an especially critical part of the clinical teacher's job. To be realistic this choice must be guided by three general admonitions:

— You don't have time to do everything that would be worthwhile
— You shouldn't select goals without consulting others
— You aren't the student's only teacher.

The first of these warnings is already very familiar to clinicians. Each day in their work with patients, clinicians must confront the disturbing fact that their potential for helping patients is seldom fully realized. Competing demands on the clinician's time, the patient's energy and the resources available to pay for health services all force unwelcome decisions about which of the patient's needs are most urgent and important, and which must be ignored or given only limited attention. The time, energy and other resources available for clinical teaching are equally scarce. Only when our students' needs are very simple and specific can we hope to meet them fully. In most cases, in order to help students achieve a useful level of mastery in the most important areas, some types of learning must be given low priority and dealt with superficially or not at all.

Clinical teachers are seldom free to set these instructional priorities entirely on their own. Other clinicians who help care for a patient may have their own ideas about what he needs to learn and how each professional discipline should contribute to his instruction. Administrators in hospitals and other health agencies usually regulate the type of new staff orientation they require and the amount of staff in-service education they will subsidize. The college and university programs from which clinical field-work students will receive their degree or certificate usually specify the areas they feel should be included in clinical assignments; and, of course, the patients, staff, and students themselves come with a variety of personal interests, concerns and ideas about what they want to learn.

Faced with these unavoidable limitations on what can be accomplished and on the clinical teacher's autonomy in selecting instructional goals, it is comforting to realize clinical teaching is not a solitary effort. Each clinical instructor adds only a limited piece to the student's overall learning. By the time students encounter the clinical teacher some of them have already learned many of the things they need to know. In selecting goals the clinical teacher must find out what the student can already do and build on this. After their formal clinical instruction is finished most students will have continuing formal and informal opportunities to learn. The clinical teacher must decide what really needs to be learned here and now and what can be postponed until later. While the clinical instructor is at work with a student many other people may also be trying to help that same student learn. The clinical teacher must coordinate what she does with the work of these other teachers to try to prevent gaps, duplication and conflict in the student's overall instruction To carry out this selection, negotiation, and coordination of goals calls for a range of skills too broad to be covered thoroughly in this handbook. Several excellent sources of additional help are suggested in the bibliography at the end of this book. The guidelines and exercises presented here will focus on only a few of the most important steps in goal setting.

QUESTIONS TO ANSWER AS YOU CHOOSE OBJECTIVES

In deciding what to attempt to do on any given day the clinical teacher must pull together the results of three very different sorts of assessment.

1. Functional assessment

This considers the role and responsibilities for which students are being educated and attempts to answer the questions:

- What tasks will this student be expected to perform in the future?
- What knowledge, skills and attitudes will he need to learn in order to do these things safely, effectively and in a way he finds satisfying?

2. Student assessment

This examines the individual student's personal characteristics to determine:

- What are this student's personal interests and concerns? What does he most want to learn? Are there things he wants to avoid?
- What has this student learned previously that will help (or hinder) his performance of expected tasks?
- Does this particular student have any special strengths or weaknesses that will influence how quickly he learns or how he learns best?

3. Situational assessment

This analyzes the specific strengths and weaknesses of the time and place in which the clinical teacher will be working with the student and compares this situation with others to ask:

- Which of the various things this student needs to learn do I have the time and resources to help him with?
- Which will he be prepared to work on when he comes to me?
- What could be done as well or better in some other time and place?

These questions serve as filters to separate out the instructional goals that are most feasible, important and appropriate for the instructor to work on here and now. This process is summarized in Figure 2.

This is a process that demands collaboration. The teacher cannot select objectives wisely if she does this entirely on her own—too many important questions can be answered only by the students or by other instructors. Exercise 4 will let you see some of the steps such collaboration involves.

Figure 2 A process for setting instructional priorities.

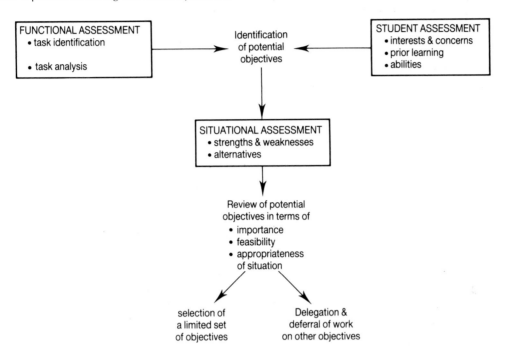

CONSULTING WITH OTHERS ABOUT YOUR OBJECTIVES

Your work on this exercise will be most interesting and useful if you can arrange to do it with a group of other clinical teachers. They do not need to be from the same professional field as you. Alternative instructions are provided in case it is impractical for you to work with a group, or if you simply prefer to work on your own.

Please allow at least 30 minutes for this exercise. The only materials you will need are a pen and several sheets of paper. If you are working with a group it will also be very useful to have a blackboard or flip chart you can use to summarize the ideas of different group members.

TASK A Form a small work group

Find at least two other clinical teachers who will work on this exercise with you. If possible, at least one of them should be from a different professional field. An ideal work group would be 4 or 5 people. Avoid groups larger than this because it will limit individual participation and make completion of Task E too time consuming for it to be interesting.

TASK B Select the patient for whom you will plan

Read the following two brief patient descriptions and decide which you prefer to imagine is the person for whom you will be choosing instructional goals. You will need to draw on past experience in completing some of the tasks, so choose the case with which you feel most familiar.

Patient A is: A 42-year-old who a week ago during a routine chest x-ray was found to have a non-calcified, non-encapsulated nodule in the apex of the left lung. The patient entered the hospital this morning and is scheduled for pulmonary function tests this afternoon and an exploratory thoracotomy tomorrow morning for suspected left upper lobe cancer.

Patient B is: A 23-year-old secretary who fell while running to catch her bus on the way to work several days ago. In the fall she suffered bruises of both knees and dislocated her right shoulder. She was admitted to the hospital and had a successful closed reduction of the dislocation. X-rays show no fractures, but the arm is still stiff, sore and swollen. Her general medical work up showed her general health status is good; however she also discovered she is now two months pregnant.

TASK C Decide the role of each group member

If you are working with a group, each of you will be asked to think about goals from a different point of view. Assign each member one of the following roles:

— *the patient*: one person should take the role of the patient you selected in Task B. You may decide privately on any personal characteristics you want to imagine this patient has in addition to those in the case description.

Each of the other group members should take the part of a different health professional who might be involved in teaching this patient. These might be:

— a staff *nurse* on the patient's unit who will have principal responsibility for his/her care today
— a *dietitian* assigned to this area of the hospital who ordinarily sees each patient early in his/her stay
— a *clergyman* or woman from the clinical pastoral counseling staff of the hospital who stops to see the patient because he/she checked on the admission form that such a visit would be welcome
— a *physical therapist* who has been asked to see the patient by the physician.

If you wish, you may substitute another type of health specialist (e.g. social worker, pharmacist, medical technologist, etc.) so long as it seems reasonable for that person to have contact with this patient today and to have some concern for teaching the patient about his/her health and health care.

If you are doing this exercise alone, begin by taking the part of the patient. After you have completed Task D from the patient's standpoint, shift your thinking and draw on your clinical experience to do Task D a second time from the standpoint of a professional staff member.

TASK D **List your instructional priorities**

Work independently *without* discussing your ideas with the other members of your group.

If you are taking the part of the patient, imagine that you are alone in your hospital room and that so far you have had very little opportunity to ask questions or discuss your health problems and health care with anyone on the staff. *Write a list* of things you would like to have a health professional explain if they were available for half an hour to do this now. When you've written down all the things you'd like to know, go back and put a star * in front of the three things that seem most important to you personally—the things you would like to be sure are covered if there isn't enough time to talk about everything on your list.

If you are taking the part of a professional, assume that you have not worked with this patient before, but that you will be seeing him/her soon in his/her hospital room. Your schedule will allow you to spend not more than half an hour talking with this patient and teaching him/her about health and health care. *Write a list* of the things you would like to teach this patient today. Then go back and put a star * in front of the three things you feel are most important—the ones you want to be sure to get to if there isn't enough time to go over everything.

TASK E **Combine your lists**

If you are working in a group, the easiest way to do this is to make a chart on the blackboard or flip-chart. Make a column for each group member and place their lists side-by-side on the chart. State the person's role at the top of the column. Start with the people who took the parts of the professionals. As each person reads out their list, write key words on the chart to describe each item they want to include. Fill in the patient's list last.

If you are working alone you can simply put your two lists on the table next to each other.

TASK F **Discuss the results**

Begin by talking with each other about anything you think is especially interesting in any of the lists or about thoughts you had as you worked independently. Then turn to the Feedback section for suggestions on additional ways in which your work on this exercise might be analyzed.

EXERCISE 4

FEEDBACK ON EXERCISE 4

The following four general questions can be used as a framework for thinking about the logic and thoroughness with which you went about setting instructional priorities for this patient.

1. *Can you justify each of the things on the professional's list?* You should be able to explain how each component of your teaching will help this patient cope with his/her present and future health needs and health care. Be especially suspicious of any plans you have to give the patient abstract scientific information (e.g. describing the food groups or naming the lobes of the lung) unless you can be quite specific about how the patient will use this information. It's not enough to simply say something vague, such as: 'The patient will feel better if he understands this.' Try not to be too strongly influenced by what is traditional in your field. Health professionals are often guilty of 'dumping' information on patients that the patients don't really need. This may help build the patient's confidence in the professional's expertise, but it uses a great deal of valuable time that might otherwise be spent on more practical matters.

2. *What assumptions did you make about personal characteristics of the patient that might have a strong influence on his/her needs for information and advice?* The brief case descriptions provided for this exercise were designed to be somewhat uninformative. Health professionals often begin work with patients knowing very little about them. As a clinician you may have seen many patients with health problems similar to those described in the case you selected. This certainly should help you to anticipate some of the needs such patients probably have in common: what their immediate health care will involve, how they might respond, and what they will need to do in order to take an active part in their own health care. However, personal characteristics may be just as important as diagnosis in determining what these patients want and need to learn at this point. For example, if you worked with patient A, did you feel you needed to know:

- whether a family member or close friend of the patient has had lung cancer?
- whether this patient or someone he/she knows well has recently had major surgery—and if so was it recent and similar enough to give the patient some idea what to expect?
- is the patient a smoker?
- does he have health insurance or other assured sources of payment that keep financial concerns from being a major worry at this time?
- what sort of work does the patient do?
- does the patient's educational background make it likely he/she has some idea what terms such as 'pulmonary function' mean?
  If you chose Patient B, did you make any assumptions about:
- whether this will be her first child?
- whether she is married?
- whether she is right or left handed?
- what recreational interests she may have that involve vigorous use of the right shoulder?
These are only a few of the things that might be important in determining what instruction would be most helpful. As a staff member you could find out about some of these things by looking at the patient's medical record. Other factors may be difficult to judge until you begin work with the patient yourself. For example,
- How emotionally and intellectually receptive is the patient at this time to information and advice about his/her health?

- Is this a person who usually feels most comfortable when he/she is fully informed and given a chance to help make important decisions, or does he/she prefer to 'let the experts decide?' If you ignored such personal factors entirely, you run a considerable risk of wasting some of your limited time on teaching inappropriate or unnecessary things. As an obvious example, little can be gained by explaining the principles of good pre-natal nutrition to someone whose chief concern is how to arrange for an abortion. On the other hand, if you spend most of your limited time gathering information on the patient, you will have little opportunity to use what you have learned, and may never get to teach some of the important things most patients with this diagnosis do want and need to learn. Compare notes with the other members of your group to see how you went about making trade-offs between information gathering and giving instruction. Are there things you all agree you need to find out before you can decide how to begin? Encourage the person who took the part of the patient to tell you what sort of person they imagined themselves to be, and whether any of these characteristics had a particularly strong influence on what they wanted to learn. If you are working alone, you may find it helpful to recall real patients you have seen who were in the same diagnostic group as the person in this case. Were these people different from one another in any ways that needed to be considered in setting priorities for their instruction?

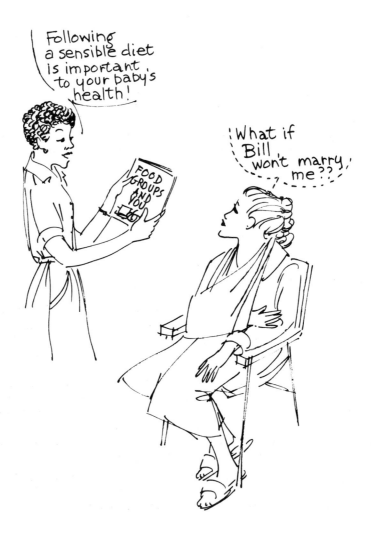

3. *How well did the needs listed by the professionals match those of greatest concern to the patient?* You can highlight similarities by drawing an arrow from each thing listed by the patient to anything on one of the professionals' lists that seems responsive. Don't worry if the words used are dissimilar so long as the intention is the same. Then look for items on both lists that do not seem to match up.

   • If the professionals are planning to teach things in which the patient expressed no immediate interest, extra work may be needed to help the patient see their relevance.

   • If the professional does not plan to respond to questions that have high priority for the patient, this also may create motivational problems. Until the patient's questions are answered they will continue to occupy much of his/her attention and may distract the patient from hearing and learning other useful things the professional does say.

   Even when the patient's questions seem unimportant or bizarre, the clinical teacher usually cannot afford to ignore them. Of course, giving a satisfactory response may be extremely difficult. In many cases the patient's most urgent questions ask for information the professional does not have or is not free to give. Such questions as:

   • Am I going to die?
   • How much will it hurt?
   • Is my doctor doing the right thing?
   • Why did this happen?

   often present such a challenge. If the people who played the part of the patient in this exercise had such topics starred on their list, discuss how you might go about explaining that you don't know the answer, or that someone else could give a better answer, without seeming frightening or evasive.

4. *Can you see any major gaps, conflicts, or duplication in the overall instruction the patient will receive if each of the professionals teaches the things they have listed?* (If you are working alone, you will need to answer this question by thinking about what other staff working with the same patient might be teaching.) If you find that several different professionals are planning to teach the patient the same thing, think about whether this duplication is worthwhile. It may help to impress the patient with the importance of a particular piece of information or advice, but perhaps the time could be used to greater advantage if one professional substituted something else. This is difficult to decide in the abstract. A more realistic approach is to begin by thinking about whether you feel confident you could cover everything on your list in the half hour available. If you could not, and if your list duplicates that of other professionals in some areas, think about what you could substitute for duplicated items? Which do you think would be most helpful, repetition or expansion of the scope of your instruction?

   Then look at the lists and consider whether in combination they will cover everything you think is important. If you find no-one in the group was planning to teach something you agree would be useful, discuss why it was omitted. If this was because none of you felt competent to deal with the topic, or you all felt restricted by professional ethics or administrative regulations, discuss how this might be remedied by seeking outside consultation, bringing in clinical teachers with different backgrounds, or seeking the authority you need to teach it yourself. If each of you left this topic off your list because you expected someone else in the group to attend to it, how might this have been avoided? Can you suggest practical ways in which the staff working with this patient might communicate with each other about their teaching plans so their efforts could be more efficiently coordinated? Try not to rely entirely on face-to-face methods of gathering and giving information. Conversations with patients and team meetings with colleagues are helpful but they also are very time consuming. Consider other methods for communication such as the problem-oriented record or interdisciplinary forms to document total instruction of patients who are taught by several different professionals.

In this exercise the focus has been on collaborative planning for patient education; however, the principles involved apply equally to staff education and instruction of professional students. There too, thoughtful setting of priorities and good communication with other teachers are essential.

FORMAT FOR STATING OBJECTIVES

Listening to students, sharing plans with other instructors and drawing upon the recommendations of experts all help the clinical teacher generate a sound list of possible objectives. However, additional work is usually needed to reduce this list to a practical length. This chapter suggested earlier that to decide which of an array of possible goals should have highest priority for a real student in a specific clinical setting the instructor must decide:

- which are most *important* in preparing this student for his probable future role(s) and responsibilities?
- which will it be most *feasible* to work on with the resources available at this time, in this place?
- which are most *appropriate* to work on here instead of during some other part of the student's total education?

Logical answers to these questions are difficult to give when the possible objectives are described in vague terms or dissimilar formats because this makes the various goals almost impossible to compare. For example, in planning for a student's fieldwork experience, a clinical instructor usually talks with the student about his interests, reviews the expectations of the student's academic program, and considers the traditions of student teaching established by other clinical staff in her department. The result is likely to be a lengthy list of possible goals described in a confusing variety of ways:

- Some may be very *global* (the school may say: 'We'd like the students to improve their problem-solving skills')
- Others may be quite *specific* (staff may agree: 'Every student who goes through this department should learn to set up patients correctly for testing on the isokinetic equipment')
- Some describe a type of *activity* that seems attractive or useful (the student may say:

'What I'd like best would be to spend time working with patients who are on dialysis')
- Still others describe *information* the students should be given (the instructor may think: 'I'll need to allow time to go over normal values for the special lab tests we use on this unit').

Further work is needed before the merits of these competing objectives can be compared. The first step is to translate them all into some sort of common terminology or format. The most reasonable way to do this is to state all the objectives by describing exactly what it is we want to help the student become able to do. Such descriptions of instructional purpose are usually called *behavioral* objectives because they spell out the type of action we want the student to learn to perform. They describe the student's behavior, not that of the instructor, just as the objectives of health care describe what the patient's future status should be, not what the health professional should do to bring that about. These objectives may also be called *terminal* objectives because they describe the behaviors we hope students will have mastered by the end of our instruction, not the practice activities that lead up to this mastery. This format reflects the definition of learning presented in Chapter 1. There we defined learning as a change in behavior. Instructional objectives, therefore, can be stated most logically by describing what we hope the end result of that change will be. The changes may take many different forms. Improved ability to remember information; new analytical, planning or judgmental skills; commitment to new values; strengthening of old interests; better performance of complex movement tasks—all may be seen as learned changes in student behavior.

In order to translate varied descriptions of instructional purpose into a behavioral objective format the instructor must be able to recognize the difference between instructional process and instructional outcome. Exercise 5 will let you test your ability to do this.

TELLING THE DIFFERENCE BETWEEN METHODS AND RESULTS

This is an individual exercise. You should not need more than 10 minutes to complete it and to check your work using the feedback section that follows. Review the objectives listed below and decide whether each one describes:

- an instructional *outcome*—something you want the student to *do* by the end of his work with you
  or
- an instructional *process*—something you want to tell the student or have him practice as a method of learning.

Write the word process or outcome in the space provided by each objective to show which you think it is.

_____ 1. The student will establish good therapeutic rapport with patients of all ages.

_____ 2. The student will judge whether a patient's maximum heart rate is within the normal range for adults of that age.

_____ 3. The student will measure range of motion in all planes at the glenohumeral joint on at least three fellow students.

_____ 4. The student will appreciate the importance of cost control in health care agencies.

_____ 5. The student will follow the problem-oriented format in making entries in the patient's medical record.

_____ 6. The student will ask her supervisor to check a draft of her progress notes before she writes them in the medical record.

_____ 7. The student will spell medical terms correctly in written communications and records.

_____ 8. The student will review Piaget's theory of development before working on the pediatric oncology unit.

————————————— 9.   The student will be exposed to more than one point of view about major issues in professional ethics.

————————————— 10.   The student will say she is interested in learning more about clinical research method.

FEEDBACK ON EXERCISE 5

You should have identified objectives 3, 6, 8 and 9 as *process* objectives. It is true that each of them describes some sort of student activity, but these are practice exercises rather than the behaviors students eventually need to master. Practicing on fellow students, having written work evaluated by the instructor and reading up on basic terms and theories all may help the student to learn, but these are methods of learning, not end results that are useful in and of themselves. Objective 9 is difficult to judge because it uses very ambiguous terminology. What does being 'exposed to' mean? In spite of its vagueness, this is obviously some sort of instructional process. It might lead to a variety of learning outcomes. The result of this experience might be:

- for the student to realize professional colleagues often disagree about important issues
- for the student to want to decide for himself which point of view he prefers
- for the student to identify the underlying assumptions and preferences that can lead to differing points of view on an issue.

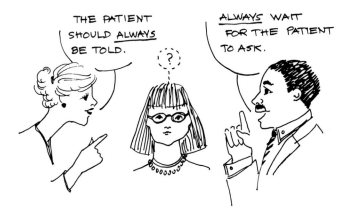

These are quite different end results. Before deciding whether 'exposing' the student to different points of view is worthwhile, or deciding just what 'exposure' should involve, the teacher needs to decide what results she hopes this experience will produce.

Objectives 1, 2, 5 and 7 all describe types of performance that could be useful results of instruction. They should have been rated as *outcome* descriptions.

Objective 4 also describes an outcome, but it uses very ambiguous terminology. What does 'appreciate' mean? Even though it is concerned with an end result of instruction, this statement is too vague to be very useful.

Objective 10 could be either a desired end result or a part of the instructional process. If your chief concern were for the student to master specific technical skills needed to design and carry out research projects, you might see this primarily as a description of useful motivation. In that case it becomes part of the instructional process comparable to reviewing Piaget's theories or practicing techniques on classmates. On the other hand, if your overall concern were to help the student acquire the professional values needed for a successful clinical career, you might regard this as a valuable outcome in and of itself. Objectives such as this may need to be seen within the overall context of program goals before we can tell whether they represent a method or a result of instruction.

OVERT AND COVERT BEHAVIOR

Stating objectives in terms of behaviors to be learned makes comparison and selection of goals easier. The instructor can examine each of the possible outcomes that competes for attention and ask:

- Will it really make a difference if the student never learns to do this?
- Can the student do this already?
- Do I have the time and resources to let the student practice this?
- What other opportunities is the student likely to have to work on this?

However, such comparison may reveal another important difference in the way different objectives are stated. Even though all describe student behaviors, some of these actions may be concrete and easily observed while others may take place without being visible to the instructor. The two types of performance are often labeled *overt* (action another person can see, hear, or feel) and *covert* (thoughts or feelings that are not observable). Calling the student's actions covert does not imply he is making a deliberate effort to keep others from knowing what he is doing, it simply means the behavior may take place without any accompanying physical action. Remembering, planning, judging, liking, fearing and a large number of other intellectual and emotional events often are covert. We can tell that someone else is doing these things only if they also say or do something overt that indicates how they are feeling or what they are thinking.

Both overt and covert behaviors are important,

and either may be the focus for an instructional objective. However, trying to help a student develop skill in a covert behavior presents a special challenge. Because the teacher cannot observe the student's behavior she cannot judge its correctness. That in turn makes it difficult for the teacher to guide and reinforce the student's practice attempts and difficult for the teacher to decide when the student has achieved an acceptable level of mastery. Some experts on instructional objectives recommend that all objectives should be written in terms of observable behaviors. This means the learned behavior itself must be overt or the objective must also include description of overt *'indicator'* actions by which an observer can tell that the desired covert behavior has occurred. We are used to relying on such indicators in our day-to-day dealings with the people around us. We judge what they are thinking and feeling by what they say, the actions they take, their facial expression and body language. Sometimes the conclusions we draw from these indicators are incorrect, but they represent the best clues we have for judging the many important covert behaviors of others. This is especially critical when we try to judge a student's emotional reactions and values — his interest, self-confidence and determination, or his doubts, fears and dislikes. In setting instructional priorities the instructor's chief concern should be simply to make sure covert behaviors are not overlooked in thinking about what students need to learn in preparation for future responsibilities. Exercise 6 will let you test your ability to tell the difference between these two types of behaviors.

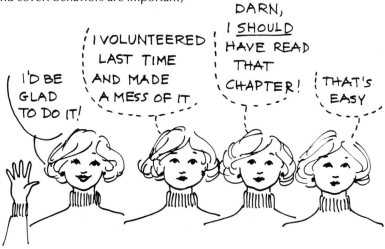

TELLING THE DIFFERENCE BETWEEN OVERT AND COVERT BEHAVIOR

This is an individual exercise. You should be able to complete it and check your work with the feedback section in less than 10 minutes. Review the objectives listed below and *underline* the word that describes the learned action or behavior that is the principal focus of the objective. This word should be a verb.

Then decide whether this verb describes:

- an *overt* action—something you or another observer could see, hear or feel the student do.
  or
- a *covert* action—something the student could do without you being able to observe directly that this was taking place.

Write overt or covert in the space provided to show which you think it is.

_____ 1. The student will spell medical terms correctly in written communications and records.

_____ 2. The student will say she is interested in learning more about clinical research.

_____ 3. The student will change a sterile dressing without doing anything that might contaminate the wound.

_____ 4. The student will recall the age at which normal children usually begin to use abstract terms as part of their spoken language.

_____ 5. The student will judge whether a patient's maximum heart rate is within the normal range for adults of that age.

_____ 6. The student will feel empathy for patients with expressive aphasia.

_____ 7. The student will measure carotid and radial pulse rates accurately.

_____ 8. The student will approve of departmental procedures designed to reduce unnecessary expenditures for health care.

_____ 9. The student will address adult patients as Mr, Mrs or Miss rather than by their first name unless the patient requests otherwise.

_____ 10. The student will set realistic objectives for long-term care of patients with progressive disorders.

FEEDBACK ON EXERCISE 6

Compare your answers with those shown below.

overt	1.	The student will spell medical terms correctly in written communications and records.
overt	2.	The student will say she is interested in learning more about clinical research.
overt	3.	The student will change a sterile dressing without doing anything that might contaminate the wound.
covert	4.	The student will recall the age at which normal children usually begin to use abstract terms as part of their spoken language.
covert	5.	The student will judge whether a patient's maximum heart rate is within the normal range for adults of that age.
covert	6.	The student will feel empathy for patients with expressive aphasia.
covert & overt	7.	The student will measure carotid and radial pulse rates accurately.
covert	8.	The student will approve of departmental procedures designed to reduce unnecessary expenditures for health care.
overt	9.	The student will address adult patients as Mr, Mrs or Miss rather than by their first name unless the patient requests otherwise.
covert	10.	The student will set realistic objectives for long term care of patients with progressive disorders.

The behaviors in 1, 2, 3 and 9 are overt because someone other than the student can observe these actions directly. If objective 1 had simply said 'The student will spell medical terms correctly' that might have been considered covert, since a student could think about how to spell a term without the instructor being able to observe that thought process directly. By adding the specification that this will be done in writing an action that could be covert is made easy to see.

In objective 9 the student's actions are easy to observe. However, we might question why this is worth worrying about. Objectives that describe learning in terms of strict 'rules' of observable behavior often seem arbitrary or unimportant unless they also manage to explain what underlying skills or values these observable actions reflect. For example, the value of this objective would be easier to judge if it said 'The student will show respect for the social customs of her individual patients by addressing them . . . etc.' 'Respecting' the preferences of others is a covert behavior, and it may seem vague or ambiguous until we are given at least one example of how this feeling might influence observable action. Neither the covert feeling nor the overt indicator taken alone provide enough information for us to judge whether this is an objective to which we want to give high priority.

The behaviors in objectives 4, 5, 6, 8 and 10 cannot be observed directly. For some such as 4, 6, and 10 it is not very difficult to think of ways to find out what the student is thinking. We could ask them to tell us, look at their notes in the medical record, or infer their judgments from the therapeutic actions they take. The covert behaviors in objectives 6 and 8 are more elusive.

They involve the student's attitudes or ways of feeling about things and if we ask about these directly the student's reply may tell us what they think we want to hear rather than what their feelings truly are. If we wanted to reword these objectives to make the behaviors overt we would need to describe indicator actions that occur spontaneously rather than 'on demand' so that we could believe they were authentic reflections of the covert emotions we really care about. For example, objective 8 might be restated, 'The student will demonstrate approval of departmental procedures designed to reduce unnecessary expenditures for health care by following these procedures consistently without being reminded'.

Finally, what about objective 7? It was marked both overt and covert because the measurement skill involved consists both of a motor performance we can easily see and a judgmental process that is not directly observable. We can see whether the student places her fingers over the correct area to palpate the pulse. We can see whether she seems to be taking the pulse for an appropriate period of time. However, unless we ask her to do something extra such as counting out loud or writing down the rate so we can see it, we cannot tell whether she is actually feeling anything or whether her counting of what she feels is correct. Many evaluative procedures have this mixed overt–covert composition. It may not always be necessary to spell out both components, but in selecting objectives and evaluating learning it will be important to remember both components are there.

GOAL ANALYSIS

All this work on restating objectives and analyzing the behaviors they involve can seem time consuming and tedious to a busy clinical teacher. Certainly objectives do not always need to be written down in polished form, and analysis of the covert and overt elements of performance often can be done very informally. Instructional objectives have no particular value in and of themselves. However, it is wise to remember why we bothered thinking about them in the first place. Setting priorities is difficult if the possible goals are vague and cannot be compared logically. Negotiation with students and other teachers is impossible if we are unable to communicate our ideas about what we think needs to be learned so others can understand what we are proposing.

The ability to describe and analyze learned behaviors is especially important when the student is trying to master a complex skill. As Chapter 1 emphasized, many of the skills we teach in the clinic actually consist of a combination of different types of behavior.

- Sometimes a student can already do many parts well, then analysis can let us focus our objectives on mastering the remaining steps.
- Sometimes the entire sequence of steps is unfamiliar to the student, then analysis can help us break it into manageable parts for early practice.
- Sometimes instructors are in the habit of beginning instruction in a complex skill by giving the student a great deal of abstract theoretical information as background. This may have little interest for the student until he can see its relevance to the tasks for which he expects to be responsible. Analysis of the tasks can help the instructor link information to the steps in performance it supports; and in many cases it can show us that some of the information we planned to present isn't really needed at all.

Goal analysis is simply an orderly procedure for deciding what specific things we need to help a student learn to do in order to prepare him for a particular job or role. It usually includes the following steps.

1. *Job analysis.* We begin by naming the major activities or tasks for which we expect the student will be responsible. For example, if the student is the mother of a normal newborn child the tasks for which she will be responsible may include such things as bathing the child, nursing it, keeping track of the baby's weight gain, bringing it to the pediatrician for vaccinations and so forth.

2. *Task description.* Key tasks are then described to say in general terms what they involve and under what conditions they will be performed. Examples might be:

   - Women who have had a mastectomy need to do self-examination of their remaining breast at least once each month, at home, without being reminded.
   - Social workers employed by institutions providing long-term care for patients who are mentally ill or retarded need to cope constructively with occasional angry complaints from families about such things as the patient's dress, cleanliness, recreation, or nutrition.
   - When a clinical pharmacist is assigned to cover the house telephone in the central pharmacy office of a teaching hospital he will be expected to answer urgent questions from the medical staff and house officers about possible drug interactions.

   Notice that these are real tasks at which the student will be expected to be competent. The student must do more than simply recall facts and procedures, he must put this knowledge to use in a practical fashion.

3. *Task analysis.* In this step we describe the series of actions someone must go through to perform the task correctly. Some steps will be overt, others may be covert, and some may involve a combination of observable action and invisible judgment or feeling. Even complex tasks usually have a skeleton of quite standardized actions that need to be performed in a particular sequence. Where some degree of choice exists in what to do, this can be reflected in the analysis by listing the principal options or by stating the conditions under which alternative actions are appropriate. For example, in bathing a newborn, a standardized step would be to test the water with your own elbow in order to judge whether it is at a comfortable temperature. If the bath is too hot or too cold, the next step is obviously to add hot or cold water to adjust

it appropriately. If the temperature is all right this step can be omitted.

To complete the analysis it is useful to classify each step as overt, covert or mixed. This helps ensure important covert steps are not overlooked. Look at Exercise 6 if you are not sure how to do this.

4. *Analysis of probable learning needs* of the category of students to whom the teacher expects to teach this task. At this point the teacher must rely on her past experience with such students, information available about their formal education and life experience up to this point, and her own logical guesses about what they probably can and cannot do. The analysis is only tentative. It incorporates many broad generalizations and suppositions. However, it still can provide a useful starting point for planning an approach to teaching the task.

The literature of education is filled with interesting and elegant systems for classifying different types of learning. Several sources of such taxonomies are listed in the bibliography at the end of the book. Such detailed classifications can be useful in studying how learning progresses from one level to another and in thinking about the relationships between different types of learning within a hierarchy of objectives. For this analysis, however, the clinical teacher can use a very simple system of classification, one that has immediate practical application to the business of planning instructional activities. Its purpose is to predict what general type(s) of learning is still needed for most students to perform each step in the task correctly. We assume the students in this category are usually not yet able to perform the entire task correctly when we begin work with them. Analysis attempts to generalize about which component abilities the students already have, and about the general nature of the missing pieces in their mastery. Each step in performance of the task should be assigned one or more of the following learning needs' classifications:

Recall — If the student probably doesn't know that he is supposed to do this, how the step should be performed, when it fits into the sequence, or under what conditions it should be included or omitted from the task.

Execute— if knowing what to do isn't enough and learning to perform will require additional mastery of new movement skills or intellectual processes. Imagine yourself telling the student exactly what to do and when to do it. If you think he still would be unable to perform the step correctly without practice, the student needs to learn execution skills.

Value — if knowing what to do and being able to do it are not enough to ensure that the student will perform the step conscientiously and with the necessary care or confidence. This classification indicates a need for learning new or stronger attitudes or feelings related to some part of the task. It is most often used for steps in performance that students may find unpleasant or intimidating, or for steps they probably don't yet see as important enough to bother with.

None — if the student probably already knows that this step is part of the task, and also knows when and how to do it, can execute the step satisfactorily, and has the necessary attitudes to do it appropriately on his own. This means you do *not* need to worry about teaching this step yourself.

5. *Identification of probable instructional priorities*

The task analysis can now serve as the basis for selecting the things this category of students probably needs to learn most. These can then be listed as objectives which are likely to be of special importance.

The heart of this lengthy process is the task analysis—a specification of all the steps a complex procedure involves. The following sample shows just how thorough and specific a good task analysis should be.

SAMPLE TASK ANALYSIS

Procedure for drawing a 5 ml blood sample from an adult patient using a vacutainer

Steps in performance	**Type of action**
1. Introduce yourself to the patient and check his/her identity by by asking him/her to state his/her name. On in-patients also check identification bracelet.	(overt/covert)
2. Explain the purpose of your visit.	(overt)
3. Talk briefly with patient to determine past experience with this procedure and assess level of anxiety.	(overt/covert)
4. Ask patient which arm he/she prefers you use, and obtain permission to examine venepuncture site.	(overt)
5. Have patient sit or lie down with arm supported and expose site.	(overt)
6. Continue talking with the patient while using finger palpation to check for a suitable site in the antecubital area.	(overt/covert)
7. Decide whether site is suitable.	(covert)
8. If suitable, monitor patient's expression and continue conversation while quickly attaching needle to vacutainer holder and placing 5 ml vacutainer tube in holder. Do not engage tube and needle. Do this without waving the needle needlessly in front of the patient.	(overt/covert)
8A. If site *not* suitable, ask to check the other arm and repeat steps 6 and 7. Then do step 8.	(overt/covert)
9. Place assembled vacutainer, alcohol, dry gauze and tourniquet on the side of the patient from which blood will be drawn. It should be within easy reach but out of the patient's direct view—to one side.	(overt)
10. Minimize patient's anxiety by assembling materials quickly, maintaining occasional eye contact and continuing conversation.	(overt/covert)
11. Tie tourniquet on upper 1/3 of arm so you can easily untie it with one hand.	(overt)
12. Instruct patient to open and close fist several times as you palpate vein for increased pressure, estimating its depth and diameter.	(overt/covert)
13. Cleanse site with 70% isopropyl alcohol and dry with gauze. Site should be recleansed if contaminated by repalpation.	(overt)
14. Explain to patient what he/she may feel and allow him/her to watch procedure or look away. (A person's reaction to a procedure often is related to how they control their anxiety.)	(overt)
15. Pick up the vacutainer assembly with your dominant hand, holding the barrel between your thumb and last three fingers with your index finger resting against the hub of the needle.	(overt)
16. With your free hand, support the patient's arm at the elbow, leaving your thumb free to compress and stretch the soft tissues below the puncture site to anchor the vein and pull it taut during needle insertion.	(overt/covert)
17. Anchoring the back of your fingers on your dominant hand against the patient's arm, insert the needle (bevel up) to enter the vein with a single, direct puncture of skin and vein. Be careful not to exit on opposite side of the vein.	(overt/covert)
18. Change the vacutainer assembly to the other hand and hold it firmly in place.	(overt)
19. Gently push the vacutainer tube forward using the flange of the vacutainer holder until the tube is engaged with the base of the needle.	(overt)

20.   Hold assembly in place until tube is filled with blood. Then   (overt)
        smoothly disengage tube from the needle and remove it from the
        holder.

20A.   If blood does not enter the tube, slightly pulling back the needle   (overt/covert)
        may help. If still unsuccessful, palpate needle and vein, then
        carefully adjust needle until blood flows.

21.   Address patient's reactions by asking, 'How are you feeling?' and   (overt/covert)
        stating, 'It's almost finished'.

22.   Release tourniquet.   (overt)

23.   Withdraw needle, and cover site immediately with a piece of sterile   (overt)
        gauze. Apply pressure over insertion site.

24.   Place vacutainer assembly and blood sample out of the patient's   (overt)
        direct view while assuring the patient that the procedure is finished.

25.   Continue to compress site until bleeding stops, then apply a small   (overt)
        bandage over the area and ask the patient to leave it in place for
        the rest of the day.

26.   Label the blood sample.   (overt)

Based on a task analysis by Loretta Donald MSN

Several features of this sample merit special comment.

First, the procedure it outlines is obviously quite standardized. In working with real patients the clinician often encounters problems or special circumstances that call for significant modifications in basic techniques. This analysis could be expanded to include additional steps concerned with judging whether the standard procedure is appropriate, and for making needed modifications when they are called for. Or this could be considered as a separate though related task, and analyzed separately. Because incorporating such decisions would make the sample analysis very long, and because modifications in technique are often not taught until after students have mastered the most frequently used form of a procedure, only the basic sequence was analyzed here.

The analysis is also notable because it includes a mixture of technical steps needed to draw the blood sample, and steps concerned with giving the patient explanations and reassurance. These could be considered as two different tasks and analyzed separately. Especially since explaining and reassuring are a significant part of so many other technical procedures, they may be tasks to which we wish to give undivided attention. They were combined in this sample analysis because of a fear that if interaction skills and technical procedures are taught separately at the outset, the student may never really combine them with the consistency we want. Rather than risk having a graduate perform a procedure with technical skill but with indifference towards the needs of the person at the other end of the needle, it seems best to analyze these different components of performance as a single integrated whole.

Because drawing blood is a physical procedure, almost all the steps listed have an overt component. However, many steps also call for some type of judgment or interpretation on the part of the professional. These components are covert. Identifying the points at which decisions are needed can help you plan instruction that takes this aspect of learning into account. In some tasks many key steps may be entirely covert.

Finally, setting priorities always involves important and somewhat uncertain assumptions about the students. For example, in this analysis assumptions might include:

• Because they have already had didactic instruction in this procedure in school, most students should be able to recall the series of steps it involves and how each should be performed.

- Because they have not yet practiced inserting a needle for this or any similar procedure, and because this requires both motor skill and confidence, work on the insertion step will be especially important.
- Although they have practiced locating a suitable vein on classmates, doing this on real patients who may be elderly, obese, or have problems that make the vessels difficult to palpate, will be quite different. Developing skill in this step with a variety of patients will be very important once the basic procedure has been mastered.
- Because they have not yet had much experience interacting with patients, and because they still will need to pay close attention to technical aspects of the procedure in order to perform it correctly, the students may forget to give the necessary explanations and reassurance or do these only half-heartedly. These will need special emphasis in early practice if they are to become an automatic part of the student's performance.

Thinking honestly and explicitly about our assumptions is a healthy part of the process of selecting objectives. It allows us to move efficiently from the task analysis to the other two types of assessment that are needed for our planning to be realistic. Throughout this chapter we have emphasized the need not only to be selective in deciding which objectives will probably be most *important* for a particular type of student, but also the need to evaluate individual students to find out whether their actual needs and concerns match our expectations, and to assess the situation in which we teach to decide which objectives it will be most *feasible* and *appropriate* to work on here and now. By identifying assumptions that have a strong influence on our probable priorities, we can pinpoint those things that it will be most valuable to emphasize as we evaluate the student and think about the types of learning experiences we are best equipped to provide.

Exercise 7 will allow you to practice using the approach suggested here by doing a task analysis of your own. Exercise 8 will let you practice building on the analysis to predict student learning needs and set instructional priorities for teaching performance of this task in a specific clinical situation.

DOING A TASK ANALYSIS OF YOUR OWN

You can do this exercise alone, with a partner, or with a group of other clinical teachers. Whichever method you choose, you will be asked to do the first draft of a task analysis by yourself. To get feedback on your work you will need to exchange your analysis with your partner or other group members. If you are doing the exercise alone you will find it most helpful if you can arrange with one other person to look at your analysis and comment on it even though that person has not done an analysis of his/her own. Alternative instructions are provided for all three feedback options.

Allow at least half an hour for your independent analysis and another half hour for discussing it with others.

The only materials you need are a pen or pencil, some scratch paper and the worksheet attached to this exercise. However, if you are working with a group, it will be easiest to exchange ideas if you have a blackboard or large piece of paper on which you can write a single master analysis that combines your separate lists.

TASK A **Make preliminary plans for the focus of your analysis**

As preparation for explaining your interests to the colleague(s) you ask to work with you on this exercise, think about your own preferences for:

- the *type of task* you would like to analyze—try to think of several that interest you.
- the *type of 'students'* to whom you might want to teach this task. These might be patients who share a common clinical problem, staff involved in an in-service program or students on a fieldwork assignment. Think about which group interests you most and at what stage in their lives you would like to think about teaching them (e.g. newly diagnosed diabetics, or staff who have worked in the department for at least a year).

TASK B **Arrange for someone to review your analysis**

If you are working with a group an ideal group size would be 3 to 6 members. You should all have similar enough clinical backgrounds and teaching experience so you will all be comfortable analyzing the same task and thinking about teaching it to the same type of students in the same sort of clinical setting.

If you are working with one partner try to choose someone who has had experience teaching the same type(s) of students as you, and who has worked in a similar clinical setting. However, comparison of your analyses will be most interesting if you work with someone whose point of view may be different in some respects to your own. If you have a choice do NOT choose as a partner someone you work with every day.

If you are working alone the person you ask to review your task analysis does not need to be a clinical teacher, but should be someone who is able to perform the task you plan to analyze. You may need to describe the type of students you teach and your instructional setting before asking for this person's comments.

TASK C **Select and describe the task you will analyze**

If you are working with a partner or group discuss the preferences you identified in Step 1 and choose a single task, type of student and teaching situation you all agree to use as the basis for your analyses. The task should be one that:

- all of you have performed at least several times and all or most of you have done recently (within the past several months)
- these students will be expected to perform as part of the role for which you are preparing them
- involves a series of different steps, many of which follow a fairly standardized sequence, at least in the basic form of the procedure.

You may also want to pick a task that is of special interest for some practical reason. It might be something you teach very frequently, or something students often find difficult to do, or perhaps one that will be a particularly important part of the student's future responsibilities. These qualities will not only make the exercise more interesting, but also may let you get ideas from the exercise you can apply to problems in teaching your real students.

If you are working alone consider the preceding guidelines for group choice of a focus. Be sure to check your plans with the person you ask to review your analysis to make sure he/she feels comfortable commenting on this task.

Fill in the task, student and situation descriptions at the top of the analysis worksheet attached to this exercise.

TASK D **List the steps in correct performance of this task**

Work by yourself on this. Use a piece of scratch paper to make a list of the sequence of things someone must do in order to carry out this task correctly. Remember, you should be describing the way a skilled person does this, under the real conditions in which the task is usually performed. Do not describe what students might do as practice activities to try to improve their abilities in this area.

Especially if this is something you do often yourself and perform easily, you may need to make a special effort to analyze exactly what your performance includes. As we gain skill in a procedure even the most difficult steps may become almost automatic. In particular you may make judgments or assessments that are important covert steps in the performance, yet not be really aware you are doing this. You might begin drafting your list of steps by simply imagining yourself or someone else going through performance of the task. However, you may then want to check your list for completeness by actually trying to perform the task exactly as you described it. If you have omitted important steps this often becomes apparent when the written list is put into action.

When you think your list is complete, write it in the left-hand column of the attached worksheet.

- Begin the description of each step with an *action verb*—something that pinpoints what the person *does* at this step
- Keep the descriptions short, but try to make them *specific* enough so another person reading your list could visualize the performance that is taking place
- List the steps in the *order* in which they usually occur
- When a step is contingent upon the results of a preceding step, show this by using an *'if . . . then'* format (for example: *'If* the water is too hot, *then* add cold and retest temperature')
- If a step can be performed in any of several different ways, show this by using an *'or'* format. (For example: *'If* A is heavier than B, add a weight to B *or* take one away from B').

EXERCISE 7

TASK E **Classify the type of performance each step involves**

In the second column of the worksheet write

overt   after each step that is usually performed through an action a observer can see, hear or feel.

covert   after each step that can be performed without this action being observable to another person.

combined   after any step in which some aspect(s) of performance are observable but others probably are not (steps that combine physical movement or speaking with some type of judgment or feeling. For example, looking at the ankles to check for swelling).

   Ignore Column 3 on the right hand side of the worksheet for now. You will need it only if you go on to do Exercise 8.

TASK ANALYSIS WORKSHEET

Task analyzed _____

Situation in which will be performed once learned _____

_____

Type and level of student, staff member or patient/family member to whom task is to be taught _____

_____

Steps in performance	*Type of Action*	*Need to Learn*

FEEDBACK

FEEDBACK ON EXERCISE 7

When you have finished your independent task analysis, give it to the colleague(s) who agreed to review it for their comments and feedback. *If you are working with a group* take advantage of the fact that you may have viewed this task quite differently from one another. One way to see differences in approach and help each other fill in gaps in your analyses is to use a blackboard or large sheet of paper to pool your ideas into one master list. Start by having one person in the group write his/her list of steps on the board. Be sure this person leaves space between steps for additions. Then, go around the group asking each member to propose *additions* from their own list and to suggest ways of *rewording* the description of any steps they feel are unclear. As you do this, also encourage group members to point out any steps they feel are unnecessary and should be *deleted*. Revise and add to the master list as you go along. Continue this until the group has reached general agreement that the list of steps is:

- complete
- clearly described
- includes nothing irrelevant.

Then compare the way you classified each type of performance. Discuss any differences of opinion reflected in your ratings in column two on the worksheet. If you are undecided about whether a step is overt or covert, ask several members of the group to actually *do* that step. If you cannot easily see, hear or feel what they are doing, the step is probably covert. If they don't all seem to do the same thing, think about whether the actions you see are really the step in performance you care about or simply some other action that serves as an observable indicator of a covert emotion or judgmental process. For example, you might want the person performing a task to 'decide what time it is'. Deciding is a covert action. They might show you that they have made this decision by saying, 'it is eleven o'clock now', or by writing the time down, or by nodding their head if someone asks them if it is 11 o'clock. These actions are all overt and easy to observe, but unless they are a normal, useful part of task performance they really don't belong in the analysis. Most complex tasks include some important covert steps. This means an observer can't really *see* another person do all the things the task involves. This is a problem for a teacher because it means she/he can't be entirely sure whether the task is being performed correctly, and can't easily reinforce the covert steps. Sometimes teachers cope with this by assuming that if the overall performance seems to go well, the covert steps must be being done correctly. At other times the teacher may feel she needs to ask the student to add something to the usual performance to make it easier to tell what thought processes or feelings it includes. The most common method of doing this is to ask the student to 'think out loud' by interjecting such questions as: 'How did that feel to you?' or 'Why did you do that?' Our emphasis on telling the difference between overt and covert actions in this exercise is intended to help you remember what these terms mean and to encourage you to regard both types of behavior as important. The chapter on evaluation includes further work on these concepts.

If you are working with a partner begin your review by exchanging worksheets and reading each other's analyses. Then put the two worksheets down side by side and compare them in detail. Discuss:

- differences in the steps that are included. Can you make one more *complete* list by combining your two analyses?

- descriptions of any steps that are unclear, or not *specific* enough so you can readily visualize the action they involve. Try to help each other reword any descriptions that are vague or use ambiguous terms. Pay special attention to the verbs. They should describe specific actions.
- any steps that may not really be *necessary*. Try to prune these out.

When you are satisfied with your lists of steps, go on to compare the way you each classified the types of performance this task involves. Please look at the instructions for doing this with a group and follow a similar process for review of your overt–covert–combined ratings.

If you are doing this alone the feedback you get from someone else will probably be limited primarily to comments on the clarity and completeness of the steps you listed for task performance. Ask the reviewer to think about how they believe this task should be performed and to read your list. Then ask for their reactions to the following questions:

1. Do you have trouble figuring out what I mean by any of the steps I've listed? Could you imagine someone actually doing what I've described?
2. Do you think my list of steps is complete? Have I left anything out?
3. Do you think everything on my list is necessary? Could someone do this task correctly if they left out any of the things I've described?

As you ask for the reviewer's reactions, be sure that person understands you are trying to describe how the task *should* be performed by someone who already knows how to do it—not how students may perform it, or how they should be taught to improve their performance. To help them do this you may need to explain at the start what sort of person you want them to imagine is performing the task, and in what type of situation you expect they will need to be able to do this. For example, if the task were 'taking medications correctly', you might need to explain you are trying to describe this task as it should be performed by 'an elderly patient, living alone at home'. If the task were 'interviewing patients and their families to determine their preferences for discharge planning', you might need to explain you want to describe how this should be done by a social worker in a community hospital.

Use the feedback you get from the review to revise your analysis until you both feel it is acceptably clear and complete.

Unless the person reviewing your analysis happens to be familiar with the concepts of overt and covert behavior, or unless you and the reviewer want to take time to go over the way the terms are defined in this handbook, you will probably need to assess your own work on classification of performance. For ideas on how to do this, please read the last section of instructions for feedback for people working in a group. You may find it easiest to take a fresh look at your own ratings if you put your analysis aside for a day or two before you attempt to rethink the overt–covert–combined ratings you wrote in column two of your worksheet.

ASSESSING STUDENT STARTING LEVEL

The task analysis you completed for Exercise 7 provides a logical framework for determining what students still need to learn. It tells us what specific types of starting level skills we need to evaluate, and makes our assessment of student needs more efficient. Usually we begin this assessment process by *predicting* what *most* students of this type already know when they reach the point in their overall instruction at which we will be working with them. Then we go on to test at least the most important of these predictions by trying to find out whether they fit the *individual* students we will actually teach.

Predictions about probable starting level are usually based on two types of information:

- our own observations of similar students we have taught in the past
- descriptions of other instruction such students have received.

If we are very lucky we will have copies of the instructional objectives other teachers working with these students have used as the basis for their teaching. If these are not available we must find out what we can about the types and amounts of instruction the student has probably been given, and do our best to guess what knowledge and skills this may have let the student acquire. Sometimes the information available is skimpy indeed. For example, the physical therapist who teaches patients with sprained ankles how to use crutches may know only that the staff in the emergency room usually explain a little about why crutches are necessary before the patient is sent to physical therapy. The nursing supervisor responsible for training new staff to work in the pediatric intensive care unit may know only the general outline of topics covered in orientation for all new employees, and a little about the amount of emphasis on intensive care procedures in the curriculum of the local nursing school she herself attended. In such circumstances the clinical teacher would be sensible to invest time in learning more about the other training her students received. Meanwhile, the importance of checking the students' actual starting level is obvious. This can be done in any or all of several ways. The instructor can:

- *Ask the student* to assess and explain his own level and needs. This is an important part of the process of 'contracting' with students to arrive at an instructional plan which they have a major role in designing for themselves. However, if the tasks the student will be expected to perform are still very unfamiliar to him, asking for such self-assessment may be futile.
- *Test the student* by asking him to attempt to perform the task so we can judge his level of mastery for ourselves. If done formally such testing can be both intimidating for the student and time consuming for the instructor. However, sometimes assessment can be incorporated without fuss into the initial teaching process. Especially if the instructor begins by asking the student to do a few things that will probably be done correctly, this can encourage the student by showing him he already has some mastery of the tasks at hand.
- *Use evaluations made by other teachers.* Sometimes these are available as formal grading reports for students or performance evaluations for staff. Documentation of patient education often includes written notes on which skills a patient appears to have mastered or appears to still be having problems with. At other times the only way to get these evaluations is to talk with the other instructors by phone or in person. Many clinical teachers are uneasy about knowing how other instructors have evaluated their students, fearing that this will bias their own judgment and make them treat students unfairly. This risk is greatest when the other assessments are very global and speak mostly of general ability or motivation. More specific evaluations are far easier to check for yourself, and help students gain recognition for what they already know. This aspect of 'fairness' to students should not be overlooked.

Exercise 8 asks you to do several of the steps needed for a learning needs assessment related to the task you analyzed in the preceding exercise.

DOING A LEARNING NEEDS ASSESSMENT

If you have not already completed Exercise 7, please begin by doing that. This exercise is based on the Task Analysis you completed for this earlier exercise.

As in Exercise 7, you will begin this exercise by working independently, and then be asked to show your work to at least one colleague to get feedback on it. If possible, do this exercise with the same individual(s) as for 7. To complete this exercise you will need the task analysis worksheet you used in Exercise 7 and an extra sheet of plain paper.

STEP 1 **Predict the probable learning needs of this type of student**

Work by yourself to review the student description at the top of the worksheet and to think about what steps in the task students in this category may already have learned to perform. What sources of information could help you make these predictions? Have you worked with many of these students before? Do you have access to descriptions of other parts of their usual training in areas that might have relevance for this task?

Summarize your predictions by filling out column 3 on the right-hand side of the worksheet. Opposite each step in performance write as many of the following ratings as you think appropriate for the *average* student in the category you are considering.

Recall — if most students don't know yet that this step is supposed to be part of performing the task, or don't yet know how the step should be performed or when it should be done. This means they still need to learn to recall some or all of these things.

Execute — if most students would still be unable to perform this step correctly even if you told them exactly what to do. This means they still need to learn execution skills.

Value — if most students probably still need to learn different or stronger ways of feeling about this step. The term value is used very broadly to show they still need to learn something such as self-confidence in performing the step, or willingness to do it even when this is difficult or a nuisance.

None — if you expect most students already have learned all they need to about this step. This means none of the types of learning represented by the other three ratings will be needed.

STEP 2 **Describe some practical things you could do to assess an individual student's actual starting level**

Still working on your own, review the learning needs ratings for the 'average' student you made in Step 1.

● Choose one step in the task for which you rated the average student's learning needs as *none*
● Choose any two other steps you felt most students would *not have mastered fully* at the time you begin work with them.

On a separate sheet of paper write short descriptions of practical things you could do in your own work situation to find out whether an individual student is at the level of mastery you expected for each of these three steps in task performance. Be as specific as possible in explaining what types of information you would want and when and where you could get it.

For example, you might plan such steps as:

1 'Before my first meeting with the patient I would ask if anyone in his family has ever been on a low sodium diet'.
   or
2 'Before the new staff member arrived on the unit for orientation I'd call personnel to ask whether she has worked with terminally ill children before.'
   or
3 'During the first few days the student is assigned to me I'd have him assist me with several aphasic patients so I could see whether he tries to use any non-verbal techniques for helping them communicate.'

Choose the method that you think would

- be easiest for you to use *and*
- at the same time would give you really accurate information about this student's present mastery of this specific step.

If you find it possible to combine assessment of several factors in a single information-gathering method, please feel free to do this.

FEEDBACK ON EXERCISE 8

As in Exercise 7 you will need to rely on one or more of your professional colleagues to help you evaluate the thoroughness and logic of your work.

If you are working a group or a partner

Begin by comparing your ratings of the types of learning most students will probably need. Discuss your individual reasons for giving ratings on which you disagree. Such differences might exist

- because the level of the students with which you have worked in the past has been different. In your own work settings some of you may teach this task to students with little prior training, while others teach students in the same general category who have a lot of earlier preparation.
- because your standards for acceptable performance differ. The task analyses didn't spell out how well each step must be performed in order to be acceptable. If your standards for this differ, one of you might say the students probably have nothing left to learn while another instructor would say they probably still need further work on recall, execution and/or values.

Use this exchange of ideas primarily to help you decide whether your own predictions seem *realistic* to other clinicians.

Then compare the sources of information you each have available to help you with these predictions. Pay particular attention to ways in which different people feel they can find out about the other training that students in this category receive. Use this comparison primarily to find out whether you have *overlooked* any sources of information you might actually be able to use.

Finally, compare the different techniques you used to evaluate individual students' actual starting level.

Use the following questions to help you compare the methods you used:

1. Which method is most *practical*? Which takes the least time and is the least likely to be disruptive for you, other staff, and the student?
2. Which is most *timely*? Which will give you the information you want early enough for you to take maximum advantage of this in planning for this student?
3. Which is likely to provide the most *accurate and specific* information about the student's present mastery of this particular task?

Unfortunately these qualities don't always go together. You may need to make trade-offs. For example, many clinicians who supervise student fieldwork customarily ask each new student to write a short statement for them listing what the student feels are his/her own major strengths and weaknesses at this point and suggesting some of the things on which he/she would most like to work during this assignment. This is certainly practical for the teacher, and it does leave the student free to express his/her own interests and priorities. However the student's statements are often far too global to be terribly useful in deciding what the student's present level is in relation to mastery of specific tasks. For some students this may also seem like a rather fruitless guessing game in which they must try to figure out what the teacher wants them to want to learn. Such global self-evaluations can indeed be a useful starting point for learning about individual students, but if this is the only technique you planned to use you probably should consider adding at least one more specific method of evaluating competence.

If you are working alone

You will need to rely for feedback on someone who has not done this exercise himself. Begin by reading the suggestions for group feedback to get ideas you can use in reviewing your own work. Then

- show your worksheet to a colleague who knows how to perform the task and who has had some contact with this category of students. Ask this reviewer whether he/she thinks your ratings of the average student's *probable* starting level are realistic.
- Then show the reviewer your plan for evaluating an individual student. Ask if he can think of any other practical ways you might find out about the student's level; and if he can suggest
- any other methods that might be easier, more timely, or provide more accurate information.

The principal purpose of this review is to help you get new ideas from other clinicians on how to predict and measure student needs. You will not be looking for 'mistakes' in your own work so much as trying to pick up things you may have overlooked and looking for better or easier ways to do this important part of goal setting.

SITUATIONAL ANALYSIS

The final step in this marathon process of selecting instructional objectives is review of the individual teacher's instructional resources. Feasibility and efficiency are of particular concern. This review should show the instructor which goals she is especially well equipped to help students achieve, and which could be achieved more easily somewhere else. An instructor may decide not to work on an important objective for any of the following reasons:

- if it is still too early in their education for students to accept the need for this sort of learning
- if they have not had the necessary preparation to practice the skills involved safely and productively
- if she herself lacks the breadth and depth of expertise needed to give accurate direction and feedback
- if the facility doesn't have the space, equipment or programs needed for the students to actively practice the skill
- if administrative procedures or rules make student participation in a practice activity difficult
- if the instructor and others will not have time to provide the supervision and feedback needed.

Even when none of these obstacles are present, a wise instructor may decide not to try to help students with some objectives simply because another instructor in another setting could do an even better job.

Because clinical instructors often work with students at a point very near the end of their overall education, deciding on the best time and place for work on objectives may be difficult. When a patient is already drowsy from pre-medication and knows someone is on the way to take him to surgery, it is obviously not a good time to try to teach him breathing and coughing techniques. Yet if this is the only time the nurse or therapist can reach him, she must try to make the best of a poor situation. If a student is due to graduate in a few weeks, and his clinical supervisor discovers he still has not learned an essential skill that logically should have been taught early in his education, she too will have to do the best she can. However, the logic of situational analysis need not be totally wasted even in such discouraging encounters. It can still be used to try to change the system so that future students will receive instruction in an appropriate setting and at a favorable time.

Situational analysis calls for skills in planning instructional sequences and in assessing the resources needed for effective use of different teaching methods. Later chapters in this Handbook provide suggestions for how this can be done. At this point we will only point out the practical importance of asking yourself at regular intervals:

'Which of these objectives can I really help students achieve?' and

'Could the student learn this more easily somewhere else?'

UNRESOLVED ISSUES

This chapter has recommended an approach to instructional planning that is frugal, analytical and pragmatic. It values wise use of time, collaboration with others, and teaching based on logical planning rather than custom or whim. However reasonable these guidelines may be, they still leave unanswered many important questions concerning instructional priorities. Consider, for example, the following concerns:

1. Shouldn't all teaching help the individual student grow as a person, learn about himself, and explore things simply because he's interested in them instead of putting so much emphasis on preparation to perform practical tasks? Isn't this a narrow and technical view of education?
2. If instructional activities are all planned in detail before you begin, won't this make them very rigid? Will the instructor be willing to abandon or change a plan in which she has invested a great deal of effort if the plan doesn't work? Won't this make instructor and student ignore and waste wonderful opportunities for learning simply because they weren't expected when the plan was made up?
3. How cut-and-dried are the responsibilities for which our students need to be prepared? Isn't one characteristic of a profession that the tasks performed are usually not routine?

4. How far into the future should planning extend? Should students be prepared for the things we know they will be expected to do now, or for things they may be expected to do in the future? Professional practice and health care technology are changing rapidly. How can the teacher guess at what patients or professionals may need to do in the future? Shouldn't education try to create changes as well as respond to change?

Honest discussion of any of these questions calls for consideration of philosophical and practical matters that go far beyond the scope of this introductory Handbook. However, these are not issues even the beginning clinical teacher can afford to ignore. The position you take on issues such as these will have an immediate and very pervasive effect on many of the practical choices you make in your day-to-day teaching. Because my own present point of view on these questions inevitably colors many of the guidelines suggested in this Handbook, some of my opinions are summarized briefly here. Reading them may help you interpret recommendations in other sections of the book. More important still, I hope they will provoke you to think further about your own point of view on these issues. This is perhaps the 'ultimate exercise' for a teacher. For feedback you will need to rely on frank discussions with your students and with fellow teachers and keep an honest eye on the real world consequences of following the philosophy you adopt.

Here then, some opinions on instructional priorities in clinical teaching:

1. Most clinical teaching is initiated for very practical reasons. Patients, other staff and students seek (or tolerate) our instruction because they believe we can help them learn to do useful things. Competence at these practical tasks often has a major effect on the patient's future health and sense of well-being, the staff member's effectiveness and the student's ability to get a job. We are not free to ignore practical objectives in deciding what we will teach.

2. Even within the framework of very practical training, instructors can provide rich opportunities for students to explore their own interests, exercise independence and learn about themselves. By allowing instructional options that match different learning styles, and using the many resources for experiential learning available in the clinical setting, instructors can help students invent and test their own techniques, discover their own solutions to practical problems and build their own sense of identity as they do these things.

3. Work on such personal growth objectives is most likely to receive the attention it deserves if these goals are as clearly defined as those for scientific and technical competence. An inarticulate belief that students should have opportunities to chart their own course and grow as people is difficult to implement and is easily endorsed but then ignored.

4. Most practical tasks can be performed safely and effectively in more than one way. Students should be encouraged to identify options and to examine those options critically in terms of their consequences and logic. Instruction should be designed to teach students to be suspicious of rigid rules of performance that are supported only by tradition or by the charisma or authority of the person who endorses them.

5. However expert the instructor may be in deciding what her students need to know, this help is available to the student only on a temporary basis. The student's future needs are almost sure to be different from those of the present. Before formal instruction is ended the teacher must help the student learn to assess his own needs, set his own priorities and locate his own resources for continued growth.

Think about your own point of view on these issues.

3 IMPROVING MOTIVATION AND COMPLIANCE

Nothing is more disheartening to a hard-working teacher than a student who doesn't want to learn—except, perhaps, the student who learns obediently but then ignores all we have taught once he is on his own. The first of these problems we label lack of motivation; the second, non-compliance. In both, the element of student 'willingness' is critical. These problems remind us that it is the student, not the teacher, who controls learning. Of course, learning can be imposed by a teacher who is sufficiently clever and determined; and students often learn from experiences neither they nor the teacher have planned. However, the sensible teacher depends more on planning and persuasion than on good luck or coercion in getting students to learn and do the things she believes are worthwhile.

THE NEED FOR ACCURATE DIAGNOSIS

When we find a student is ignoring our instruc-tion, simply repeating our original lessons and exhorting the student to try harder may be futile. We must try instead to unravel the many different forces that could interfere with the student's 'willingness' so we can attack the problem at its roots. One systematic method for doing this instructional detective work can be borrowed from the many analyses of health behavior conducted in recent years in the field of Public Health.[1] The models developed through these studies recognize that accurate information is only one of the things that must be provided in order to promote sound health practices. They focus attention on the ways in which an individual's beliefs, values and resources influence his willingness to translate information about recommended behaviour into consistent action. To see how this analytical model might be applied to finding the causes of a compliance problem, try applying it to your own health behavior by doing Exercise 9.

ANALYZING YOUR OWN HEALTH BEHAVIOR

You can do this exercise alone. It will take about 15 minutes.

In 1972 Belloc and Breslow[2] from the University of California in Los Angeles published the results of a major study of the relationship between health status (life expectancy and illness) and compliance with six commonly recommended health behaviors. These behaviors were very broadly defined and included:

1. eating three meals a day, including breakfast
2. maintaining body weight within ± 10 pounds of normal for your age, sex and height
3. getting regular physical exercise
4. having 8 hours of sleep a night
5. drinking alcohol only in moderation or not at all
6. not smoking.

TASK A

Begin this exercise by thinking about your own level of compliance with these six recommendations during the past 6 months.

Summarize your evaluation by writing one of the following ratings opposite each recommendation in the compliance column of the attached worksheet.

Usually: if you have followed this recommendation consistently during the past six months; done this on all but a few unusual days.

Occasionally: if you have followed the recommendation at least 30% of the time, but can't honestly say you have done this consistently.

Seldom: if you have rarely or never complied with the recommendation during the past 6 months.

TASK B

Now review any of the behaviors for which you gave yourself a rating of 'occasionally' or 'seldom' to think about *why* you have not been complying with these recommendations consistently. If you *do* usually follow all six recommendations, shift your analysis and think instead of a family member or close friend whose behavior you know well and who does *not* comply fully with one or more of the recommendations. What might be contributing to their actions?

Summarize the results of your analysis by writing one or more of the following key words in the probable cause(s) column of the worksheet opposite each recommendation followed only seldom or occasionally.

- Lack of *information*: if you didn't know this was recommended by many experts, or if you knew it was something you should do but didn't know how.
- Lack of *conviction*: if you aren't personally concerned about the health problem(s) this behavior is supposed to prevent, or don't believe the behavior really is effective.

- Lack of *opportunity*: if you believe this is worth doing, and know how, but don't have the time, money or other resources you need, or aren't free to do this because of restrictions imposed by other people.
- Lack of *net benefit*: if you could do this and feel it might be helpful to you; but believe what it would require you to give up is worth more to you than what you expect you would gain.

Use the bottom section of the worksheet to make notes on specific things that lead you to give these ratings, and to describe any factors different from those listed on the worksheet that were important to you in deciding whether to follow these recommendations.

EXERCISE 9

HEALTH BEHAVIOR ANALYSIS WORKSHEET

Recommended behavior	Compliance rating	Cause(s) of non-compliance
1. Eat 3 meals daily including breakfast		
2. Keep weight within ± 10 lbs of normal		
3. Get regular physical exercise		
4. Sleep 8 hours a night		
5. Drink moderately or not at all		
6. Don't smoke		

Notes on specific reasons for any failure to do these things consistently during the past 6 months.

FEEDBACK ON EXERCISE 9

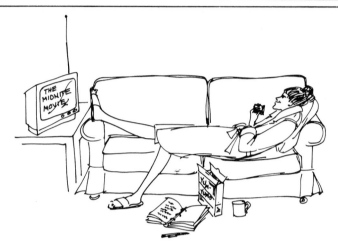

To see how this sort of analysis could be used to improve compliance, think about what it would take to get you to change your health behavior. Consider the possible causes of poor compliance and the types of interventions each seems to require for correction.

Lack of information can be a serious obstacle to good health practices. However, most adults in industrialized, Western countries have probably been told they should do these six things since childhood. Parents, teachers, the mass media, even relative strangers all are likely to have recommended these actions at some time. Moreover, the recommendations require little special skill or instruction to follow. However, despite their familiarity, you might have found these very general recommendations difficult to follow without more specific guidelines. What does 'regular exercise' mean? Which of several different height/weight tables should you use? What must you eat in order for this action to count as 'a meal'? Without such key pieces of specific information you may have felt these recommendations were too vague to convert into actions. If you recorded lack of information as a cause for your own imperfect compliance in Exercise 1, take a moment to think about exactly what type and amount of information you would need in order to improve. Such selective planning for instruction is important for any teacher faced with a compliance problem.

Lack of conviction that following a recommendation would be useful might be the result of any of several different types of belief. The Health Belief Model proposes that an individual will be unlikely to take a recommended action to avoid a health problem unless he holds three beliefs:

- that he is *susceptible* to the problem
- that the consequences would be *serious* if the problem occurred, and
- that the recommended action would be *effective* in preventing it.

Consider whether your own inconsistent compliance can be traced back to a problem with any of these basic beliefs. Breslow and his associates found that among the white, male Americans they surveyed, those who complied with five or six of the recommendations had a life expectancy 11 years greater than subjects who complied with fewer than three. Differences between the two groups in their rates and patterns of illness were equally impressive. Although you may never have heard of this particular study before, you probably have seen some objective evidence in support of many of the six recommendations. Unfortunately, that does not guarantee you believe the actions are worthwhile for you. You may feel that although many people do need eight hours of sleep you really feel better with less. You may feel the effectiveness of some practices hasn't really been proven. ('For every expert who says smoking causes cancer I'll show you another who says it doesn't.') Or, you may believe trying to ensure your health by following this set of recommendations is futile, since they cannot offer comprehensive protection. ('What's the use? I knew someone who did all these things religiously and was killed in an automobile accident when he was 34.') Since in the uncertain world of health care few actions can be absolutely guaranteed to produce a specific effect, doubts about the significance of recommendations may be difficult to overcome. If you recorded lack of conviction as a possible cause of any of your own non-compliance, try to decide exactly what type and amount of evidence someone promoting these recommendations would have to present in order to convince you to follow them. Would statistics about the experience of others be convincing—or would you need to see some objective evidence that you are personally vulnerable to a specific health problem? Would you need a chance to test the action on a trial basis to see whether it made a significant difference for you, or might a thorough and logical explanation be enough to convince you? Any effort to change your behavior by changing your beliefs would be most likely to succeed if it were focused directly on your specific areas of doubt.

A perceived *lack of net benefit* may be a more common cause of non-compliance with these six recommendations than is complete lack of belief in their value. Our concerns about health must compete with a wide range of other interests. We are reluctant to follow recommendations that are unpleasant, demanding or embarrassing. We are especially unlikely to do things that require us to give up immediate satisfactions in the uncertain hope of avoiding a possible problem in the distant future. You may recognize that you don't exercise because you find it boring; argue that it's pointless to give up smoking because you will only gain weight, or believe it would do serious damage to your career or your social life if you went to bed early enough to get eight hours sleep. Any improvement in your compliance in such situations would depend on your perceiving a significant change in the balance between gains and losses. If lack of net benefit was a factor in your Exercise 9 ratings, consider which strategy seems most likely to be feasible and effective: one designed to strengthen your belief that the recommended action would be beneficial, or one that emphasized helping you avoid or cope with associated losses?

Lack of opportunity to follow a recommendation exists when the barriers to action are external rather than related primarily to a lack of knowledge of what to do or a belief this would be worthwhile. For example, if you have a wakeful new baby who needs attention throughout the day and cries and fusses for hours most nights, you probably have little opportunity to follow the eight hours of sleep recommendation. For the six recommendations that are the focus of Exercise 9, external barriers probably are not a major cause of non-compliance for most health professionals. However, when we try to analyze the sources of non-compliance in our patients and students we may want to begin by making sure they have the time, materials and support from others they need to do what we recommend.

Reflection on your own health behavior may have shown you that your compliance with some recommendations results chiefly from factors that have nothing to do with health. You may exercise because you enjoy it, watch your weight because you care about your appearance or avoid alcohol because of religious beliefs. When such related preferences support the teacher's recommendations they make compliance easy to achieve; but when they work in the opposite direction they may block even our most determined efforts to convince students our recommendations are worthwhile. Certainly our efforts to strengthen willingness and reduce obstacles to action must take into account many different aspects of the student's life, not simply those that are our immediate concern in teaching a specific behavior.

The most important conclusion to be drawn from this exercise is that efforts to improve compliance must be directed towards removing the causes of the problem if they are to succeed. Little can be gained by giving someone information on how to do something for which they see no need. Equally little will be accomplished by trying to make someone worry about a problem if they don't know how to solve it.

STEPS IN DIAGNOSIS

Evaluating the reasons for our own occasional lapses in recommended behavior is fairly easy. We are close enough to our own knowledge, beliefs, resources and constraints to be able to pick out major obstacles when they exist. However, analyzing the reasons for non-compliance among the staff, students and patients we teach may be difficult—particularly if their life style, level of knowledge and situation are very different from our own. Then the teacher must try to put herself in her student's place, and attempt to imagine what that person knows, values and is free to do. The student who has only recently begun professional training as a dietitian may find the detail of a required course in biochemistry boring because she has no idea how it can be used in her future work with patients. The arthritic problems of middle age may seem unreal to a 13-year-old who detests the orthopaedic shoes she is told to wear. A salesman may be uneasy about taking pills during a business lunch even though this seems routine to the health professional who recommends it as a way of reducing gastric irritation from a needed medication. A sensible teacher can guess that such obstacles need attention, but these ideas about possible cause should be carefully tested before they are used as the basis for remedial action. Diagnosing the causes of poor compliance in others calls for three quite different steps:

1. The clinical teacher should begin by *describing the performance problem* in clear, concrete terms. Something makes us uneasy about the student's behavior, but what? Exactly what is the difference between what the student does and what we have tried to teach him to do? Is he not doing something often enough? Doing it incorrectly? Not doing it at all? Or is he persisting in doing things we have recommended he avoid? We must specify the nature of the problem before a logical search for its cause can begin.

2. Then the teacher can review what she knows about the student to *make a preliminary guess* at what may be causing the poor compliance. What specific knowledge, beliefs and resources does the recommended action require? By comparing these with what she knows about the student's past instruction, apparent abilities and concerns, and by thinking about the student's probable responsibilities and support system, the teacher can often arrive at some tentative conclusions about obstacles that need attention.

3. Because this initial diagnosis often is based on very subjective or fragmentary evidence, the teacher should *systematically gather further information* to explore and test her initial ideas before planning a remedy for the problem. This may call for further observation of the student, review of records or discussions with colleagues, formal testing, or simply sitting down with the student to discuss concerns, obstacles and alternatives.

Exercise 10 will let you practice this three-step process with a sample case.

DIAGNOSING THE CAUSES OF PATIENT NON-COMPLIANCE

The instructions for this exercise explain how it should be done by a group of clinical teachers during a one hour in-service class or workshop. You can do the exercise alone or with only one or two other teachers by skipping or adapting the tasks that call for exchange of ideas with other participants. However, be sure to do Task E *before* you begin to compare your ideas with those in the feedback section of the Handbook.

TASK A **Read the four case problems**

Quickly review the attached cases to decide which one you prefer to analyze for this exercise.

TASK B **Join a group of participants interested in this case**

Go to the meeting area in which everyone interested in the case you chose has been told to assemble. (The person responsible for practical arrangements for the class should tell you this.) Form a work group of from 4 to 6 members.

TASK C **Work by yourself to begin analyzing the case**

Before you begin to discuss the case with the other members of your group, please take at least 10 minutes to work independently and do the following:

1. Re-read the case carefully and circle or underline any parts of it that you feel tell you the patient's compliance is unsatisfactory or doubtful.
2. Write a sentence or two at the top of the attached worksheet to describe the compliance problem as you see it. Summarize exactly what the patient seems to be doing wrong or failing to do.
3. Review the information you have about this patient to see if you can make some preliminary guesses about why the problem exists. Go down the *determinants* in the *compliance checklist* on the attached worksheet and think about whether any of them might be responsible for this patient's non-compliance. To record your evaluation on the worksheet:
   - Check *OK* for each determinant you feel probably is present to the degree needed for compliance
   - Check *not OK* if the factor seems to be lacking and if you think this may be interfering with compliance.
4. Finally, use the bottom section of the worksheet to outline a plan for gathering additional information that would help you test the soundness of your checklist ratings.

   On the left side of the page make a list of questions you feel need to be answered before you decide how to try to improve the patient's compliance. On the right side of the page make a note telling where or how you might get the information you need. For example, on the left you might list: 'Has the Dr told the patient his diagnosis?' and on the right note: 'Check the Drs note in the record' or 'Ask the Dr at rounds tomorrow.'

TASK D Exchange ideas with the other members of your group

Use whatever process you prefer for telling each other about your independent analyses, but try to make sure that each member of your group has an opportunity to say what he thinks and take time to explore differences of opinion.

By the time you finish the discussion, please:

- Compare your problem descriptions to see whether they all have the same focus
- Tally the groups' ratings to see how many people checked *OK* and how many *not OK* for each determinant
- Make a master list of the questions your group agrees need to be answered to test your initial diagnosis and of your practical plan for getting the information you feel you need.

If you find you don't all agree on any parts of the analysis, allow time to discuss *why* you have different ideas about the case.

Finally, choose one member of your group to be your spokesman when you compare the way different groups analyzed each case in a general discussion at the end of the class/workshop.

TASK E Keep track of general questions and ideas you want to explore

One purpose of this exercise is to help you identify aspects of compliance you would like to discuss with other teachers. You may want to ask for advice on how to interpret a problem you encounter frequently or may want to sound out others on their reaction to an approach you feel is helpful. It will help to make notes on these topics to remind you of points you want to raise in discussions today or to explore through your own reading and conversations with other teachers in the future.

TASK F Discuss the exercise with the class as a whole

As with the discussion in your small group, the purpose of this session is to compare approaches, raise questions and share ideas on practical methods you have found useful in getting at the causes of compliance problems among your own patients. Broaden the discussion to include compliance problems among staff and students if you wish. The same general approach to diagnosis should be useful for all three groups.

When you have finished this class you may want to review the additional comments provided in the feedback section of this workbook.

CASES

Case A

Alice Mahoney is a 68-year-old woman with chronic obstructive lung disease. Five weeks ago she was admitted to the intensive care unit of your hospital with pneumonia and in respiratory failure. She was tracheotomized on admission and was on mechanical ventilation and oxygen with frequent endotracheal suctioning for several weeks. Mrs Mahoney is now improved, and was recently weaned from the respirator and her tracheostomy closed. Last week she was transferred to an intermediate care unit in the hospital where she is currently being maintained on nasal oxygen.

This patient is alert and friendly, but appears very apprehensive. You have taught her to do breathing and coughing exercises and have explained she needs to do them frequently throughout the day to keep her lungs clear. You also have encouraged her to sit up in the armchair next to her bed several times each day and to begin walking around her room to build up her general endurance. She is badly deconditioned from her illness and long stay in intensive care.

Staff on the unit have agreed that major goals for Mrs Mahoney are to improve her activity tolerance and ability to clear pulmonary secretions sufficiently for her to be discharged to the three room apartment she shares with her husband. Joseph Mahoney, a 71-year-old retired carpenter, visits his wife daily and seems eager to have her return home as soon as possible.

Although Mrs Mahoney does her exercises well when you are with her, and can walk short distances without support, when you look in her door on your way to see other patients you usually find her in bed asleep or watching television. Staff on the unit are concerned because they have had to suction Mrs Mahoney to help her clear her airway several times each day since her transfer from intensive care.

Case B

Betty Masters is a 16-year-old secondary school student who lives in a suburban town with her parents and two younger brothers, Andrew, aged 12, and Ralph, 11.

A year ago Betty was diagnosed as diabetic after complaining for several months of unusual fatigue. Her diabetes now is well controlled so long as she follows the special diet she was taught in the diabetic clinic.

Betty is a bright, outgoing girl who seemed to have little difficulty learning the diet when you explained it to her. She appeared to really understand such concepts as food groups and exchanges, and was able to apply these to a selection of appropriate foods. She did equally well at learning to test her urine. As part of your instructional program you offered Betty several booklets published by the Diabetes Association explaining some of the basic things patients should know about the nature of the disease and the rationale for its treatment. Betty took these home to read, and commented to you later that they were interesting.

This morning, when she came in to the clinic with her mother for a 6 month check-up, Betty's blood sugar values were slightly abnormal. On careful questioning she admitted that she hadn't been 'doing too well' with her diet. 'You don't understand', she complained. 'After school all my friends go down to Bob's Ice Cream for a chocolate shake or a sundae. They'd think I was creepy if I said I just wanted a piece of plain fruit or something. I don't want them to think I'm some kind of invalid.'

'The worst is in the mornings', her mother added with resignation. 'Betty spends so long putting on all that make-up; and then she rushes down and says she hasn't got time for breakfast. Usually she just grabs one of her brother's doughnuts or a sweet roll and rushes out. I know she doesn't always take time to test her urine either.' 'Well,' replied Betty, 'I don't see what all the fuss is about. I feel fine now.'

Case C

Arthur Bullock is a 4-year-old cerebral palsy patient with moderately severe athetosis. He was referred to you 2 months ago when his family moved to your area because his father, an electrical engineer, changed jobs.

Because he has poor head and trunk control, Arthur has been given an adapted wheelchair that provides good lateral and posterior support. He has never been ambulatory.

Although psychological testing shows Arthur has normal intelligence, his speech development has been delayed because of his difficulty in controlling head position and because his control of tongue, facial muscles and breathing is poor. A month ago you taught Arthur's mother a set of exercises to do at home to help him improve control in these areas. She seemed to understand the importance of getting Arthur into a good position in the chair before starting, and was able to guide him through the exercises without even looking at the set of written reminders you gave her. She agreed to do the exercises twice daily, allowing about half an hour for each session.

Because they live some distance from the hospital, Mrs Bullock brings Arthur in to see you only once every 2 weeks. Today when they arrived you began by testing Arthur's head control and breathing. Arthur tried hard to do everything you asked, but seemed to you to have made no improvement. You asked Mrs Bullock to show you what she had been doing at home while you held Dora, her 8-month-old who usually comes along on their visits. As Mrs Bullock began, Arthur started to cry and fuss. 'Oh, he does that every time I try to get him to do the exercises', she said with despair. You reassured her that it was important to keep trying, and told Arthur he needed to work hard. 'It's been especially hard this week', Mrs Bullock explained. 'His sister Mary, who's 7, has been home from school with the flu. I'm afraid some days I haven't been able to do the exercises even once.' Then she asked: 'His dad says he could do the exercises after work, but he thinks it would be better if we were working on something Arthur really wants to do—like walking. Do you think we could try that?'

Note: If you work with this case, focus your analysis on Mrs Bullock not on Arthur.

Case D

Mary Costello is a 63-year-old retired waitress who has been taking medication for high blood pressure for the past 2 years. She was divorced 15 years ago and now lives alone in a small apartment about two miles from the hospital. On previous visits to her physician her hypertension was found to be well controlled.

Today Mary came to the hospital pharmacy to have her prescription for a diuretic refilled. A check of pharmacy records showed that she should have needed a refill nearly six weeks earlier. When asked whether she had been taking her pills as frequently as the doctor ordered, Mary replied, 'Sure. I do just what it says here', and reached into her purse to produce a folded piece of green paper. It was a copy of the medication instructions she had been given when the pills were prescribed originally. The instructions had been filled in with Mary's name at the top and included the name and a description of the appearance of each pill, clear instructions on how often each was to be taken, and a short explanation of why each pill had been prescribed. The pharmacist, who was one of a team that had helped design this form, was pleased to see she had it, but was concerned enough to check her other prescriptions. Mrs Costello also was several weeks overdue for a refill of her hypertension pills. When asked if she still had some, she replied,

'Well no. I'm out of them too, but they're so expensive I thought I'd wait just a little bit longer to get more—maybe until I get my pension check next week.'

Mary was then asked to go to the medical clinic to have her blood pressure checked. It was significantly elevated and the nurse who checked it continued the questioning about the pills. 'I really try to be good about taking them,' Mary explained, 'but sometimes I get busy and forget.' 'Besides', she continued, 'if I'm doing something like going shopping with friends or to the movies I just can't take that diuretic. It's too hard to find a toilet when you're out, and a lot of them aren't very clean when you do find them.'

EXERCISE 10

A DIAGNOSTIC CHECKLIST FOR ANALYZING COMPLIANCE PROBLEMS

In Case _____ the problem with the patient's present performance is _____

_____

_____

POSSIBLE CAUSES

Rating   **Determinant**

_____OK, _____not OK   1. *Knows* what health *problem* he is expected to help prevent or correct.

_____OK, _____not OK   2. *Believes* he (or the person cared for) is personally *susceptible* to this problem.

_____OK, _____not OK   3. *Believes* the problem will have *serious consequences* if not prevented/corrected.

_____OK, _____not OK   4. *Knows* what *action* he should take, and when and how to carry it out.

_____OK, _____not OK   5. *Believes* this action *would help* to prevent/correct this problem, and believes he *can do it.*

_____OK, _____not OK   6. *Physically and intellectually capable* of doing what is expected or has the necessary assistance to do so.

_____OK, _____not OK   7. *Has* the time and material *resources* needed.

_____OK, _____not OK   8. *Feels free* to perform without being unduly criticized or causing problems for others.

_____OK, _____not OK   9. *Expects* the *benefits* of the recommended action will *outweigh* its costs.

_____OK, _____not OK   10. *Has* a practical system of *cues* to remind him when the recommended action should be performed.

PLAN FOR GETTING FURTHER INFORMATION ON POSSIBLE CAUSES OF THE PROBLEM

Questions   Sources of answers
(continue on next page if necessary)

Questions   Sources of answers

FEEDBACK

FEEDBACK ON EXERCISE 10

Problem description

As you compared problem descriptions with other members of your group you may have found they were dissimilar either because you expressed your ideas in different terms or because you drew different conclusions from the information in the case summary. For example, if you worked with Case A, you might have said the problem is that Mrs Mahoney:

- isn't doing her exercises and getting out of bed as frequently as she was supposed to do, *or*
- is afraid to try things on her own, *or*
- is letting herself remain at risk of pulmonary complications and dependency because she isn't doing what she was taught.

The first of these is in the most useful format for describing a compliance problem because it focuses on the patient's *performance* and explains how it is different from what was taught. By contrast, the second statement describes one possible *cause* of the non-compliance, and the third emphasizes its possible *consequences*. Both fail to explain exactly what flaws need to be corrected in her actions. Thinking about consequences is helpful in deciding whether a performance problem matters enough for us to try to correct it. Analyzing causes is essential in order to plan logical strategy for correction. However, these steps in analyzing non-compliance are unlikely to be useful if they are based on a vague or confused concept of the problem itself.

You may have found it difficult to be very specific about the performance problem in your case on the basis of the limited information provided in the summary. The phrases you underlined in this case description probably provided a variety of clues, but many of these may have seemed ambiguous or incomplete. For example, each case provides some evidence that the patient (or mother) is not doing a recommended activity frequently enough. However, there is little to tell us whether they are performing correctly when they do attempt to do what they were taught. Case A tells us that Mrs Mahoney does her exercises correctly when you are with her; but how does she do them when she is on her own? In B, Betty tacitly admits she sometimes skips her daily urine test, but does she do it correctly when she does take time? In each of the four cases your plan for further information gathering may need to include efforts to find out more about actual performance so all aspects of the problem can be clearly described.

Initial ideas on the cause of the problem

None of the people described in these four cases appear at first glance to lack a working knowledge of what they are supposed to do (determinant 4). All seem to have performed correctly at an earlier stage, and several have been given written instructions to fall back on if they forget what they were told. Their grasp of the reasons for these recommendations is less easy to determine. While all seem to have had some early explanation of what the recommended actions are supposed to accomplish, and why this is important, the case summaries don't tell us enough to feel sure these explanations were fully understood. You may feel you want to find out more about what the subject in your case actually knows; however other determinants probably should be of even greater concern in this initial assessment.

Case A

In Case A, for example, lack of self-confidence (5), physical stamina (7) and external obstacles (8) may all combine to account for the patient's reluctance to get out of bed more often. Can she reach her slippers and robe? Is she able to cope with detaching or transporting the nasal oxygen source? If you take care of these things automatically when you are with her you may not realize she is unable to deal with them on her own. Mrs Mahoney also may have little faith that what she does really will help make her better (5). After weeks of enforced passivity, receiving frequent and often mysterious treatment at the hands of a variety of expert professionals, Mrs Mahoney may have difficulty believing her own breathing and coughing are enough to keep her alive. It may seem safer to continue to depend on the nurses' suctioning—however unpleasant—than to risk trying to clear her airway alone. You might have labeled this as a lack of information (1 or 4) rather than a lack of confidence in her own actions. Certainly it is an example of one of the many points at which lack of information and lack of confidence or motivation may go hand in hand.

Another quite likely cause of Mrs Mahoney's infrequent practice of the breathing and coughing exercises is the lack of periodic reminders that they should be done. Although she knows what to do, she may simply lose track of time and forget to exercise. Without the usual rhythm of familiar activities, often deprived of a watch and eyeglasses to read the time, and with the additional disorientation of frequent naps, many patients in hospitals have difficulty following a schedule. Instructions to 'Do this once each hour' may be more difficult to follow than 'Do this three times whenever there is a commercial on the TV program you're watching.'

Other explanations may be more complicated and subjective. For instance, you might suspect that Mrs Mahoney is not aggressive in her attempts to improve simply because she is enjoying the comfort of being looked after. She may not particularly enjoy the prospect of going back to caring for her husband, particularly if they have a small, cold apartment, few visitors and an antique and unreliable TV set. Or, she may feel no special effort on her part is necessary at this stage and think: 'It would be easier to wait until I feel a little stronger' or 'They expect too much of me after I've been so sick.' Such initial guesses certainly need to be carefully tested before they are accepted; but at this stage we should at least be wondering whether Mrs Mahoney is likely to believe the advantages of doing what we recommend will outweigh the disadvantages (10).

Case B

While Betty appears to have mastered the technical aspects of her home program easily, the case provides several clues that she may not be convinced of its value. For example, her comment that she doesn't 'see what all the fuss is about . . .' should make you suspect that she hasn't yet accepted just how serious the long-term consequences of uncontrolled diabetes can be (3). Although the booklets she read doubtless explained this in some detail, now that her original symptoms are better Betty may have difficulty believing those warnings really apply to her (2). If she has been very careless about testing her urine, she may have no evidence that breaking her diet has actually had any bad effect. Conversely, you might wonder whether Betty believes doing these things will have any long-term effect on what she knows is a serious disease (5). Even though the instruction she has received was optimistic, she may have read or heard things that have made her believe diabetes is in fact a powerful and incurable disease about which little can be done. Such fears may be difficult for a patient to talk about even when they have a strong influence on actions.

Perhaps most obvious of all is the possibility that Betty is non-compliant because of all the diet requires her to give up. The nuisance of having to figure out what she can and cannot eat, the need to give up some favorite foods, and the fear of being pitied or laughed at by her friends, may make compliance seem not worthwhile (10). Although she has the knowledge, skill, and resources compliance requires, Betty's beliefs may lead her to give it low priority.

Case C

Obviously, this mother needs help. External obstacles, especially a lack of time (7), seem almost certain to be at least one major cause of her problem. Expecting the mother of three young children to add an hour of new responsibilities to her daily schedule is probably unrealistic unless you also can help her find someone to take over some of her other tasks. Arthur's basic care is doubtless demanding even without the exercises, and the case summary implies that she has sole responsibility for this as well as for looking after the house, her husband and the other two children. When she does find time to do the exercises Mrs Bullock often must endure the 'punishment' of Arthur's crying (8), and, since his progress is likely to be slow even if treatment is intensive, she may find little to reassure her that her attempts are accomplishing anything (5). Even if she receives help that gives her more time for exercising Arthur, this is a case in which our efforts to build her hope and support her persistence will be important.

If Arthur's father is willing to help, and can arrange to come in for the necessary instruction, this could make a valuable difference. We will, however, need to be concerned with teaching him more than just the correct techniques. His comment on the greater value of working on walking, and Mrs Bullock's interest in trying this, suggest we have important work to do if they are to fully understand why the exercises suggested earlier are important, and what the consequences of ignoring Arthur's breathing and head control problems might be (1 and 3).

Case D

Mrs Costello's irregular compliance with her medication schedule probably is related to two very different shortcomings: her failure to use any practical system of cues to remind her when it is time to take her pills, and a lack of perceived net benefits that leads her to give compliance low priority in comparison with competing activities. Forgetting to take medications on schedule is a common failing—even when the medication is important and the patient is himself a health professional. Some patients have equally great difficulty recalling whether they have taken their pills or not. Solutions range from attempts to link the medication schedule to other 'unforgettable' events such as meals or bedtime, to placing the pills in a frequently noticed location, or arranging some system of logging or graphing daily intake. To design a method that would work for Mrs Costello we would need to discover much more about her habits, preferences and environment. The case summary tells us only enough to flag this as one probable cause of her compliance problem. Exploring the reasons why she seems to give relatively low priority to taking her medication also will require further information gathering and analysis. Her comments in the case summary about the high cost of the pills and the nuisance of having to find a toilet frequently if she is away from home after taking her diuretic remind us that she does have external obstacles to overcome in order to be compliant (8). We probably would want to try to reduce these barriers by finding out whether she qualifies for any type of outside support in paying for medications and suggesting how she can modify her diuretic schedule without skipping the pill entirely. However, this may not solve the problem unless we also find out whether she fully understands why the medications have been prescribed (1) and believes her own hypertension (2) will have serious consequences (3) unless she takes her pills regularly. Your plan for gathering further information may have included talking with Mrs Costello about any or all of these aspects of her beliefs. You may also have wanted to begin inquiring about the practicality of various methods of giving Mrs Costello more frequent feedback on her blood pressure. Could she be taught to take it herself? Could you arrange for her to have it checked frequently by someone else? These questions would concern you if you feel one reason for Mrs Costello's erratic compliance is her present inability to see any evidence that failure to take the pills has any real effect.

These are only a few of the many ways in which this sample of compliance problems might be analyzed initially. You may have identified other factors that are just as significant or interpreted the points mentioned here somewhat differently. However, by now the following general conclusions should be apparent:

FEEDBACK

- Failure to comply fully with recommended behaviors can take many different forms, and
- such flaws in learned performance may be the result of an equally wide variety of different factors.
- An initial review of the specific things the student (patient) is doing wrong and of his/her personal characteristics and situation can help the instructor identify possible causes of the non-compliance.
- However, this analysis must be regarded as very tentative and possibly incorrect until further information has been gathered to test the initial diagnosis.

Information gathering

As you review your own planning for getting more information on your case, consider to what degree you did each of the following:

1. *Try to take advantage of what others might know about the problem and its causes.* You seldom need to gather information entirely on your own. Other staff who are in contact with the patient, family members and the patient himself often can provide helpful information about frequency of compliance, the circumstances surrounding problem behavior, and practical obstacles that may need to be considered. Your planning should have included some effort to check the patient's record or confer with family or other staff to draw upon information that is already available.

2. *Plan the wording of some specific questions you will ask in requesting information from other people.* Unless you are already a skilled interviewer you may need to allow time to think carefully about exactly how you will ask for information in order to avoid 'leading' questions or questions that intimidate and put the respondent 'in the wrong'. This is especially important if you plan to gather information by discussing the problem with the patient or family. A carelessly worded question can easily lure them into telling you what you seem to expect rather than the truth of the situation, or may destroy the self-confidence they need in order to follow your recommendations.

3. *If you suspect the cause of the problem is something that could be easily corrected, test your diagnosis by trying out the solution.* Sometimes it is far easier to try to solve a problem than to gather additional information about its possible cause. This might be true, for example, if you noticed some easily removed obstacle that had been overlooked in initial instruction of the patient, or felt the recommended actions could be modified to make them easier to understand or follow. Of course, you may find that these easy 'solutions' make little difference, but often they provide useful shortcuts in an otherwise time consuming diagnostic process.

4. *Encourage the patient to work with you as a responsible partner in looking for the source of the problem.* Although the term 'compliance' implies a certain amount of obedience on the part of the patient, in the long run it depends on the patient's belief that he is responsible for his own behavior and that doing what we recommend will help him achieve something he values. Your plans for information gathering should have included some effort to invite the patients (or mother) to share their ideas on what makes compliance difficult and what might help make it easier.

SIMILARITIES BETWEEN MOTIVATION AND COMPLIANCE

The importance of student 'willingness' to act was mentioned at the start of this chapter as a key element in both motivation and compliance. However, the similarities extend far beyond this general quality. One way to examine the many parallels is to re-state the diagnostic checklist used in Exercise 10 to describe the determinants of behavior in terms of student motivation to learn rather than patient willingness to comply.

For a student to be willing to attempt to learn he must:

1. Know what sort of thing he is expected to learn.
2. Believe that in the future he will be expected to perform tasks that require this type of learning, and believe he has not yet achieved the level of mastery required for acceptable performance.
3. Believe failure to perform these tasks acceptably would have serious consequences for himself or someone about whom he is concerned.
4. Know when, where and how he might go about trying to learn what is needed.
5. Believe this activity would be an effective way for him to learn, and feel self-confident enough to attempt it.
6. Be physically and intellectually capable of performing the learning activity.
7. Have the time, assistance and access to material resources needed.
8. Feel free to attempt the activity without being unduly criticized or creating problems for others.
9. Expect what he will learn from the activity will be worth more to him than any time, effort, money or dissatisfactions it may involve.
10. Have adequate cues to remind him when the learning activity should be carried out.

This list of motivational determinants can be used in the same way as the list in Exercise 10 to diagnose the possible causes of poor motivation. Here too, the process should begin with a clear description of the student's performance, of the specific actions that make us believe he is not motivated. The checklist can then guide our thinking as we try to identify possible obstacles

and missing pieces in the student's current beliefs and knowledge. Finally, as with our initial diagnosis of the reasons for non-compliance, our tentative diagnosis of the causes of poor motivation should be carefully reviewed and tested before we invest significant time in using it to plan a remedy.

CHOOSING A REMEDY

Once we know why a student is unmotivated or non-compliant the steps needed to correct the problem are often straightforward and familiar. If the student needs more information or practice we can provide it. If cues or reminders are needed we can help to arrange them. Many external obstacles can be overcome or avoided by providing advice and support or by modifying some features of our recommendations. These tasks may not be easy, but the teaching techniques they involve are reassuringly commonplace and respected. We often feel far less confident, however, when we confront problems that appear to require a change in the student's attitudes and personal values. In this situation the clinical teacher often feels both powerless and ambivalent. We doubt both whether we have the ability to change another person's beliefs, and whether we have the right to try. When we say that someone we have been teaching is unmotivated or non-compliant, we usually mean we think they are acting in a way that is not in their own best interests. The unsteady patient who risks falling because she thinks using a cane makes her 'look like an old lady', the staff member who insists on wearing strong perfume to work even though she knows this will infuriate a supervisor who will later review her for a pay raise, and the student who insists he desperately wants to work in a local hospital after graduation yet goes skiing on the Saturday the school has arranged for regional personnel officers to interview prospective staff— all seem to be acting foolishly. If we care about them, this worries us; yet we recognize they have a right to their own values and wonder whether we should interfere.

Fortunately a wide variety of non-authoritarian techniques have been developed in recent years that can help us cope with these concerns. Used correctly, these methods neither manipulate nor moralize. Their purpose is to help students examine their own concerns and beliefs, and to encourage them to choose for themselves the values and actions they prefer. This approach to teaching requires the teacher to accept a very demanding view of how it is and is not appropriate to help. In teaching students new knowledge and skills the teacher ordinarily serves as the expert, explaining the right way to do things and evaluating the student's progress towards mastery as instruction proceeds. In non-authoritarian teaching the techniques are very different.

SOME TECHNIQUES FOR NON-AUTHORITARIAN HELPING

— If the student's actions are impulsive and he often seems to simply do the first promising thing that occurs to him without considering consequences and alternatives, the teacher can try to help by
  - creating a climate in which the student feels comfortable about examining his own actions and talking about his feelings
  - asking questions that encourage the student to think about both the possible advantages and disadvantages of an action before deciding whether to take it
  - modeling an analytical approach by sharing some of his own thoughts, preferences and uncertainties about values' issues without attempting to impose these on the student.
— If the student's actions seem to be based on an unrealistic or incomplete view of what the consequences of an action will be, the teacher can try to help by
  - asking questions that encourage the student to test the reality of his expectations by observing what actually happens when other people do what he is considering
  - suggesting practical ways in which the student might safely test out a new course of action to see how it works before committing himself fully to it.
— If the student's actions seem to be inconsistent with the values and beliefs he expresses, the teacher can try to help by
  - asking questions that encourage the student to compare his own words and actions
  - listening carefully to what the student says and repeating or restating it for the student to let him reflect on whether he is really saying what he means.

— If the student rejects behavior that seems to have many advantages because it also has some major disadvantages, the teacher can try to help by
  - asking questions that encourage the student to think of strategies for avoiding or reducing the expected problem
  - suggesting some overall system for adding up and comparing the advantages and disadvantages to make sure the problem really does justify a decision to reject this action.
— If the student is just beginning to explore his feelings about actions and issues that are new to him, the teacher can try to help by
  - allowing time for the student to think and to experiment with attempts to put his feelings into words
  - showing verbally and nonverbally that he believes this effort is worthwhile
  - letting the student affirm his values by stating them to another person without fear of ridicule or disapproval.

These are not easy things to do, especially if the teacher finds her values are very different from those the student prefers. The education and counseling literature provides an abundance of practical guidelines and training exercises clinical teachers can use to develop their skill in using this approach. Several particularly valuable sources are described in the annotated bibliography at the end of this book. The exercises that follow will simply let you sample three of the many non-authoritarian methods you might use in working with non-compliant or unmotivated students.

VALUE ANALYSIS

Exercise 11 makes use of one of a large family of techniques known as values clarification or values analysis exercises. The particular technique used here is one based on the concept of Force Field Analysis developed by Kurt Lewin.[3] It regards human behavior as a dynamic phenomenon in which decisions about what to do are determined by the balance of forces that drive the individual towards a particular action and opposing forces that restrain him. It encourages the individual faced with a specific decision to summarize his expectations and preferences in a way that makes it easier to see how the overall advantages and disadvantages of different actions compare.

EXERCISE 11

WEIGHING THE CONSEQUENCES

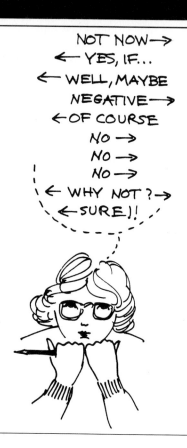

NOT NOW→
←YES, IF...
←WELL, MAYBE
NEGATIVE→
←OF COURSE
NO→
NO→
NO→
←WHY NOT?→
←SURE)!!

This exercise cannot be completed alone. You will need to arrange to do it with a partner. The exercise has two parts. In the first you will work on your own to use a structured method for describing your own preferences and expectations related to specific action. In the second part you will practice using non-authoritarian helping techniques as you work with your partner to assist each other in reviewing and expanding the analyses you began alone.

Plan to allow at least 20 minutes for your independent analyses and at least another 20 minutes for discussion of each partner's thinking. Additional time may be valuable. This is not a process that should be rushed.

TASK A **Select an action to analyze**

Try to think of some specific action you might take to try to improve your effectiveness as a clinical teacher. This might involve using some new method you haven't tried before, or simply represent changing the way you do something that is already quite familiar. The action you choose should be one that:

- you have heard (or read) someone recommend
- you believe you *could* do if you decided you wanted to
- seems to offer some promise as a means of improving your teaching
- *but* is something you aren't certain you really want to do.

Some examples might be:

— giving your patients more of their instructions in writing instead of doing this primarily by word of mouth
— meeting at the start of each day with the fieldwork students you supervise to involve them in selecting activities and reviewing their own progress
— developing a written list of the criteria you will use for evaluating the performance of staff you supervise
— or even—taking a graduate course in educational psychology.

TASK B **Arrange to work with a partner**

If at all possible, your partner should be another clinical teacher who also wants to practice this teaching technique. If such a partner is not available, try to find a co-worker, friend or family member whom you believe would be willing and able to complete all the tasks in a useful way.

In all cases your partner should be someone who:

- knows enough about the type of action you are considering and the situation in which you teach to be able to visualize consequences
- is willing to try to help you think about your preferences without trying to tell you what they think you ought to do
- is a person you feel reasonably comfortable talking with about your beliefs
- is willing to do an analysis of their own and discuss it with you.

You may find you need to modify the action decision you plan to analyze in order to arrive at something both you and your partner feel you know enough about to make a worthwhile discussion possible.

TASK C **Write a short description of the action you will analyze at the top of the attached worksheet**

Be as specific as you can. You will need to be able to visualize yourself carrying out this action in order to analyze how you feel about it.

TASK D **Make a list of the advantages and disadvantages of the action**

Try to imagine what would happen if you actually did the thing you are considering. What would this require of you and what might it accomplish? How much time and effort would it involve? How might it influence the way other people feel about you? How might it affect the way you feel about yourself? Would it be interesting? Might it be unpleasant for you—or for anyone else? How likely is it to accomplish something you care about? These are only a few of the questions you may want to ask yourself as you think about this decision. Try to consider both the tangible and the intangible consequences of the action. Try to be realistic, but feel free to include anything that might matter to *you* in making up your mind, even if you suspect other people might not agree these things are important.

Write a few words summarizing each advantage or disadvantage in the appropriate column on the worksheet.

TASK E **Rate the importance of each consequence**

So far you have simply made a list of some of the desirable and undesirable things you think might happen if you decided to carry out this action. Now you need to decide how much each of these consequences matters to you personally. How much is each likely to influence your final decision about whether to do the thing you are considering? You may want to take several different factors into account as you decide this. For example, your importance rating might be influenced by any or all of the following:

- the *magnitude* of the advantage or disadvantage you expect
- the *timing* of the effect—will it be immediate or delayed? Short lived or long lasting?
- *who will be affected*—you personally or others you care about, or will this primarily affect people you don't feel close to?
- your *personal preferences*—how much do you like or dislike this sort of thing?

EXERCISE 11

- how *confident* you feel that the positive or negative consequences really will occur.

Summarize your conclusions by using the following key to record your rating of each consequence on the worksheet.

1 = This consequence is of *little importance* to me in deciding whether to take the action

2 = This is of *some importance* to me in deciding what to do, but is only one of many things I care about

3 = This is of *great importance* to me—it will have a very strong influence on whether I take the action.

TASK F Summarize your ratings and make a preliminary decision about what to do

Add all the ratings in your advantages column. Then do the same for the disadvantages.

When you compare the two totals it may seem obvious whether you would generally gain or lose by carrying out this action. However:

- *if* the advantage or disadvantage totals are very similar
     or
- *if* you feel very uncertain about the accuracy of your expectations
     or
- *if* the numerical totals simply don't seem to 'fit' your intuitive feelings about whether to do this

you probably should give this more thought before you decide. The second part of this exercise will give you an opportunity to get help with your analysis from a partner. However, before you begin that process, summarize the results of your independent thinking by checking the decision that you prefer in the 'Where should I go from here' section of the worksheet.

TASK G Prepare for working with your partner by reviewing some of the techniques you should try to use

Begin by re-reading pages 92 and 93 in this chapter. Then turn to the 'helpfulness rating form' attached to this exercise. You and your partner will be asked to rate each other at the end of the exercise using this form. The desirable qualities are shown on the left hand side of the page, undesirable qualities on the right. Take a few minutes to think about these now, and try to keep them in mind as you try to assist your partner with her analysis.

TASK H Exchange ideas with your partner about your value analyses

This is a key step in the exercise. It is your opportunity to practice using non-authoritarian questions and comments to help another person clarify their thinking, test the realism of their expectations and choose a course of action. Your task is to support and assist without imposing your own point of view.

Decide whose analysis you will discuss first and let that partner take the initiative in starting your discussion. Allow at least 20 minutes for talking about each analysis.

TASK I Give your partner feedback on his success in using this technique

Wait to do this until you have finished discussing both analyses. Then begin by filling out the attached rating form. Put an X at the point on each scale that reflects how you felt about this feature of your partner's efforts to help. If possible, make notes of some of the specific things your partner did that you found especially helpful or unhelpful. These six rating scales describe your subjective feelings about rather general traits. Specific examples may be needed to help your partner understand why you feel as you do.

Make notes of any things that seem not to be covered by the six scales which you found important as you evaluated your partner's helpfulness. When you have completed your evaluation, exchange forms and notes with your partner. Allow time to discuss them and to share your ideas on whether you think this particular technique might be useful in your work with patients, staff or students who may be finding it difficult to decide whether they want to comply with your recommendations for action.

VALUE ANALYSIS WORKSHEET

The action I am considering taking is _____

_____

SUMMARY OF PROBABLE CONSEQUENCES

Advantages	Rating	Disadvantages	Rating

total advantages =   total disadvantages =

Where should I go from here?

_____ Forget about this change, it doesn't look worthwhile.

_____ Do this, it should be to my advantage.

_____ Try to get more information about consequences, I feel too uncertain to decide

_____ See if I can find a way to reduce the disadvantages or increase the advantages before I decide what to do.

EXERCISE 11

HELPFULNESS RATING

During our discussion of my value analysis worksheet I felt my partner's comments, questions and restatement of my comments were generally:

Clarifying ————————————————— **Confusing**

1   2   3   4   5

Helped me:

- be more concrete

- think honestly about how I feel

- see how my feelings influence my actions

- organize my thinking and put all the pieces together

For example, he/she:

Interfered with my thinking by:

- focusing on things I don't think matter

- distracting me

- making me think of too many things at once

- being too abstract & impersonal

Useful ————————————————— **Useless**

1   2   3   4   5

Helped me by:

- suggesting important consequences I'd overlooked

- giving me information I needed

- seeming to fit me and my situation

For example, he/she:

Didn't add to my thinking because they:

- just repeated what I'd said

- didn't answer my questions

- didn't seem to apply to me and my situation

Respectful ——————————————— **Disparaging**

1   2   3   4   5

Helped me feel this was worth thinking about by:

- giving me credit for having some common sense and maturity

- trusting me to follow through on my own decisions

- letting me say things my own way and at my own speed

- expecting me to be honest and being honest in return

For example, he/she:

Discouraged me from trying by:

- acting is if I were being careless or silly

- seeming suspicious or mistrustful

- interrupting me

- insisting I use other people's terms for things instead of my own

- telling me things I already know in a superior sort of way

As my partner listened to what I had to say his/her spoken and unspoken reactions seemed to be:

Attentive ——————————————— **Inattentive**

1   2   3   4   5

Encouraged me to think & talk by being

- interested

- warm

- willing to make an effort to understand

- concerned about being helpful

For example, he/she:

Discouraged me from doing this by seeming:

- bored or preoccupied

- distant or cold

- more interested in talking about him/her self than about me

Understanding	1	2	3	4	5	Misunderstanding

Seemed to interpret what I felt and said accurately by:

- picking up on the things I felt mattered

- restating my feelings accurately

- giving examples or making suggestions that really fit what I was thinking about

For example, he/she:

Seemed to ignore or distort what I said by:

- ignoring things I felt were important

- exaggerating what I said

- putting words in my mouth

- bringing up things that seemed irrelevant

Accepting	1	2	3	4	5	Judgmental

Helped me feel free to speak honestly because he/she seemed:

- open to different points of view

- willing to try to understand my point of view

- to regard me as a worthwhile person even if we disagreed strongly about some things.

For example, he/she:

Made me afraid to speak freely because he/she seemed to:

- make fun of me

- scold or threaten me

- treat my opinions as unimportant

- imply I can't be a good person if I hold 'wrong' opinions

FEEDBACK ON EXERCISE 11

The comments from your partner during Task I of the exercise will be your principal feedback on this exercise. However, as you think about this teaching technique in the future you may want to evaluate your own readiness to use it by considering some more general questions.

For example:

- In what sorts of situations do you think it would be most appropriate to use this sort of approach for trying to overcome motivation and compliance problems? When might it be inappropriate or ineffective?

- If you did decide to use this approach, how would you introduce the process to your patient, student or staff colleague? Where and when would you prefer to work on the analysis and discussion? How would you try to 'set the scene' in order to help the other person feel safe in being this explicit about their beliefs?

- How would you plan to conclude the exercise and what follow-up, if any, would you want to arrange? Would you encourage the other person to achieve closure and make a commitment to the course of action he seems to prefer—or would you rather leave this fluid? Would you feel you needed to do anything to check up on what the other person does about this in the future, or would you let it go unless he asked you for your help or advice?

These are only a few of the many practical questions that surround use of this and many other non-authoritarian helping techniques. Thinking about them should help you decide whether you are ready to try using these methods in your own teaching.

CONTRACTING

Bad habits resist change. When a motivation or compliance problem involves a long-standing pattern of undesirable behavior, even excellent informational instruction and effective programs of attitude change may not be enough to correct it. This is particularly likely to be true when the habitual behaviors are:

- highly automatic
- multifaceted or complex
- supported by some sort of immediate reward.

When this is true, the student may be unable to erase the old habit and replace it with a more desirable pattern of behavior even though she knows what she should do and truly wants to make the change. Whether the student is trying to follow a diet more faithfully, complete assignments more punctually or pay closer attention to the procedures required by her supervisor, we may hear her explain:

'I'm *trying*, but sometimes I just forget.'

'I guess I just don't have much will power.'

'Something always seems to go wrong.'

'You just don't realize how hard it is.'

Whether said in anger or in despair, such excuses remind us that many motivation and compliance problems can be overcome only by a series of small steps that whittle away at the old habit until it is gradually replaced by the behaviors both we and the student want.

Contracting is a logical technique for helping students make such difficult changes in long-standing habits. A 'contract' is simply a practical agreement, worked out by student and teacher acting as equal partners. It spells out what each will do to achieve a specific short-term goal, and usually it promises the student some sort of immediate reward for keeping her side of the bargain.

The strength of contracting lies in the fact that it:

- recognizes that major changes in behavior often need to be made little by little
- provides for reinforcement of each step in the right direction

- helps the student and teacher anticipate and avoid practical obstacles that could interfere with performance
- encourages development of an individualized plan that takes into account the student's personal style and preferences.

In the extensive literature on contracting, the rationale often is drawn heavily from research on operant conditioning. As a result, the technique is sometimes seen as simply a system for getting students to do what you want by offering them a series of small bribes. Such a focus on teacher control and on use of artificial, extrinsic rewards to shape behavior may be unavoidable if contracting is used with very young, confused or uncooperative students. However, in many cases clinical teachers can use this method to work with students, staff or patients who are both willing and able to participate as equal partners. In this case the process of negotiating the contract may be just as important as the contract itself in encouraging a change in habitual actions. If the process encourages the student to take the initiative in suggesting activities she thinks might be worthwhile, and involves her in predicting what resources and support she will need, the plan is more likely to work than if it is developed unilaterally by the teacher. Such negotiations also help to establish the student as a rational adult, capable of taking responsibility for her own actions rather than perpetuating a role as the passive recipient of praise and criticism from the teacher.

The following sample contract describes one approach to negotiating and recording a contract. Read it and then practice developing a contract of your own by completing Exercise 12.

SAMPLE CONTRACT

The performance problem

Louise Mandel is a staff physical therapist in a 300-bed general community hospital. She has worked there since graduating from the local physical therapy school 8 months ago. Her first 6 months on the job were spent in the out-patient unit, primarily treating acute orthopaedic problems. Two months ago she was rotated to the general in-patient service where her case load includes a large number of older patients with strokes, hip fractures and other problems involving some degree of long-term physical disability. Brenda McKenzie, the senior staff supervisor on the unit, is generally pleased with Louise's work. However, she is concerned about Louise's consistent failure to plan ahead for her patient's care after discharge. In her bi-weekly supervisory conferences with Louise, Brenda has pointed out some of the problems this has created for patients. For example, although Louise does a good job of teaching home exercises to family members, she often waits so long to schedule these sessions that the relatives are unable to come before the patient is discharged or must come at a time that is very inconvenient for them. Several of her patients had to spend extra days in the hospital because Louise had not yet begun teaching them specific functional skills they needed to be able to cope at home, and one patient recently had to wait for two weeks for the home health agency therapist to begin coming because Louise had failed to initiate a request for this service prior to discharge.

In these conferences Louise agreed that early discharge planning is important, but explained she gets so involved in trying to make sure the treatment she is giving at the moment is good that sometimes she forgets to take time to arrange for what her patients may need later on.

Brenda recently read an article in a professional journal about contracting and asked Louise if she would be willing to try it. Louise agreed, and they arranged to use their next supervisory conference for this.

The negotiation process

Brenda and Louise had half an hour for their conference. Brenda began it by saying, 'Let's see if we can keep this simple and agree on something that's not going to be too hard. We don't have to solve this problem all in one swoop. Can you think of a couple of different things you'd be willing to try that might be a step in the right direction?' 'Well,' replied Louise, 'one idea I had was that I could promise to talk with the social worker about each of the patients on my schedule sometime next week to see what she thinks about whether they can go home or will need to have some sort of institutional care when they're discharged. But', she hesitated, 'I don't know if I'd have time to do all that and still treat all my patients.' 'It does sound pretty ambitious,' said Brenda, 'and you might have problems getting that much of the social worker's time in one week. But let's hang onto that idea while we see what other things we can think of. Is there something you could do with just a few of your patients instead of all of them?' Louise thought a minute and then suggested, 'How about something with their functional training? I like doing that.' 'Yes, and you do a nice job of it too' replied Brenda. 'If you could focus more on finding out what skills they'll need when they're discharged that could be a good place to start. Any other ideas?' The two discussed several other possibilities such as scheduling family teaching sessions or meeting with the visiting nurse, but came back to the idea of functional training as the most promising. 'How about starting with just one type of patient', Brenda suggested. 'Why not start with the kind of patients you enjoy treating most?' 'What I'm really interested in is the amputees,' replied Louise, 'but we don't have very many. It would take an awfully long time before I got anywhere.' After a pause she went on: 'But I like working with the hip fracture patients too, and I always have a couple of them on my list. I did a paper on functional training for hip fracture patients my senior year. I could use it for ideas.' 'Good!' responded Brenda, 'I think we've got something we can use for our first contract.' They then went on to work out the following written agreement.

CONTRACT

1. *Long-range purpose* for Louise to learn to start systematic planning for her patients' discharge early enough to avoid problems or delays when they are ready to leave the hospital.

2. *Immediate goal* By the time this contract is completed Louise will have made individualized functional training plans for each of four new hip fracture patients. These plans will be documented in the patient's record within 2 days after the patient is assigned to Louise, and will describe how she expects to work on each of the self-care and ambulation skills the patient will need.

3. *Plan of action* to accomplish this Louise agrees to:
   - talk to each new hip fracture patient she is assigned, or, if necessary, a family member to find out about his/her pre-injury living situation and functional status, and about the demands of the situation to which the patient expects to go when he/she leaves the hospital
   - check with the social worker or primary nurse if these expectations seem unrealistic or unclear
   - decide what specific functional skills the patient will need for discharge and in what order these should be taught
   - write a summary of this plan in the patient's record within 2 days after she starts work with him/her.

   Brenda agrees to:
   - assign two newly admitted hip fracture patients to Louise during each of the next two weeks
   - be available to talk to Louise in the staff room between 4:30 and 5 pm each day in case she has questions about her functional plans.

4. *Contract period.* This contract will begin on March 1 and end on March 12.

5. *Plan for monitoring progress*
   Louise will: keep a log showing when she completed each step and describing any problems she has in doing this or in carrying out the rest of her schedule.

   Brenda will: check the record of each new hip fracture patient she assigns Louise to see whether a functional training plan has been documented within 2 days, and to judge whether it seems to be a complete and realistic plan for preparing for discharge.

6. *Reward and penalty.* If Louise fulfills her part of the contract, Brenda will arrange for her to leave work two hours early the following Thursday to attend a lecture on new types of artificial limbs being given at the University.

   If she fails to complete the contract Louise agrees to work one extra Saturday morning next month under the usual staff payment arrangements.

7. *Signatures*

Louise Mandel	*Brenda McKenzie*
Staff Therapist	Supervisor

February 21

Date

DESIGNING A LEARNING CONTRACT

In this exercise you will practice negotiating and writing a contract for activities to help a student take one step towards correcting an habitual performance problem. You will need to work with a partner in order to complete the tasks this involves. The instructions for the exercise use the terms 'student' and 'clinical instructor' to describe the two people who negotiate the contract. If you prefer, you may assume instead that one of you is a patient and the other a clinician, or that one partner is a junior staff member and the other her supervisor.

If you can arrange to do this exercise along with several other pairs of clinical teachers, you all may benefit from comparing your contracts at the end.

Allow at least an hour for the exercise. Before you start Task A take time to read the instructions for the entire exercise. This will help you organize your work on the component tasks.

TASK A **Choose a partner and a problem focus for your contract**

- Begin by arranging for a partner who can spend at least 45 minutes working on this exercise with you. If possible, this should be another health professional who has clinical teaching responsibilities similar to your own.
- Decide which of you will take the part of the student. If your partner is not another clinical teacher, ask that person to be the student while you take the part of the clinical instructor.
- Then select one of the following performance problems as the basis for your contract. If you prefer to practice contracting with a patient, read these examples for ideas and then develop a short problem description of your own based on habitual compliance problems you have seen in your clinical practice.

Student 1 consistently has problems keeping up with her assigned work schedule. The quality of her work is good, but she often arrives 10–15 minutes late for work, or gets to departmental meetings well after they have begun. Although her work load is the same as that expected of other students in this unit, she often spends so much time on the first jobs she is assigned that later in the day patients are kept waiting and other staff must help out to complete necessary tasks. Earlier attempts by the clinical instructor to help the student plan a realistic schedule and set priorities have resulted in only temporary improvement. 'I really feel bad about keeping people waiting and making other people do my work', the student explains earnestly, 'It's just that I get so interested in what I'm doing that I guess I lose track of how long it takes.'

Student 2 has been repeatedly criticized by the department's Audit Committee for failure to document his work with patients promptly. His clinical skills are good, and notes in the patient's records are excellent when they are finally written. However, in spite of many reminders that failure to meet the required timetable for documentation could cause serious problems for both patients and staff, the student continues to be tardy in much of his record keeping. During a recent conference with his clinical instructor the student said he realized note writing was important, but explained, 'I always seem to run out of time or get interrupted before I can get to the paperwork.'

Student 3 has good clinical skills and gets along well with individual patients, but has difficulty taking the initiative in asking questions or making suggestions, particularly when he is speaking to someone in authority or a person he doesn't know well. His clinical instructor has pointed out that this is a particular problem during staff meetings or rounds when a patient with whom the student has been working is being discussed. Although his answers to direct questions are usually adequate, the student's failure to volunteer information sometimes interferes with good team planning. In conferences with the instructor the student has said he realizes his silence must make things difficult for other people sometimes, but that he always has had trouble speaking in front of a group or with strangers.

Student 4 has been warned repeatedly by her instructor that she must be more careful about wasting expensive supplies. For example, today, while working at the appointment desk, the student used the back of a specially printed form to make a note of a telephone number, even though there was a pad of scratch paper handy. Soon after that she used a large sterile dressing to mop up some coffee another person had spilled in the staff room. When reminded about the need to control costs and conserve supplies the student apologizes sincerely and says, 'I know it's bad, but when I get in a hurry I just forget.'

These problem descriptions provide only enough detail to give you some ideas of the specific behaviors that make up the problem. You and your partner may add other details if you wish.

TASK B **Set the scene for your contract negotiations**

As you and your partner work out the details of your plan for activities to help the student overcome this performance problem, you will need to think about the practical constraints and resources available in the place where your contract will be implemented. To make sure you are both thinking in the same terms, take a few minutes to discuss and agree on the following:

- the student's professional field and level of experience

- the type of agency or facility in which you both work

- the instructor's position and supervisory relationship to the student

- other features of the setting that may have a bearing on what is and is not feasible, such as: your usual work schedules, the number and types of other students and staff who are present, type(s) of patients served, physical layout of the work area, and so forth.

Try to agree on a setting you both find easy to visualize.

TASK C **Negotiate an agreement**

Your purpose here is to think of something specific the student could try to do that would make some improvement in the performance problem with which you are concerned. Then you will need to decide what the instructor will do to help. The process you use for planning this will have a powerful effect on the value of the contract. Try to follow these guidelines during your negotiations:

- Let the student take the initiative in proposing activities he/she might attempt.

- Take time to explore a variety of ideas, don't feel you have to accept the first good idea one of you suggests.

- Don't be too ambitious. Remember, this is only the first step.

- Be realistic. Think carefully about what each activity would involve for each of you.

- Keep your plan simple. Avoid activities that require complicated arrangements, special resources, or that may be disruptive for other people.

- Try to start with a success. Pick something both student and instructor feel confident in attempting.

- Keep the discussion positive. Don't spend time complaining about or apologizing for past problems. Concentrate on finding a practical way to make improvements.

As you plan, think about each of the topics listed below. Use whatever method you prefer for keeping track of your ideas. When you reach a final agreement, summarize it in writing on the attached contract form.

Components of the agreement

1. Long-range purpose

The problem summary described some of the things the student has been doing wrong. To provide a positive framework for your planning, begin by talking in general terms about how the student will perform once the problem has been corrected. The sample contract on page 106 provides an example of such an overall description of long-range purpose. Once you agree on this, have the student write a short description of your long-range purpose in his/her own words.

2. Immediate goal

Now consider what specific change you both think would be a realistic first step towards your long-range goal. Here you will need to think in terms of a much more modest achievement.

- If the long-range goal calls for a number of different changes in what the student does now, you might begin by trying to make only one or two of these.

- If the long-range goal involves doing something very frequently, you might start by trying to increase just a little.

- If the long-range goal is for the student to voluntarily perform tasks that are unpleasant, difficult or threatening, you might begin by attempting to do this type of work under conditions that are relatively supportive.

Whatever you choose for this initial attempt at improvement, be sure you describe what the student should accomplish in specific enough terms so that you will both find it easy to judge whether the effort was successful.

3. Plan of action

This is the real 'nuts and bolts' section of your agreement. It explains exactly what each of you will need to do in order to achieve the end result you described in your short-range goal. Usually it works best to begin by thinking about what the student will do. Then, consider what, if anything, the instructor needs to do to make those student actions possible. Take time to explore several different types of activity. Let the student's preferences guide your choice unless this places unreasonable demands on the instructor or creates problems for other people.

When you have reached agreement, each of you should write your part of the bargain on the contract form. Be sure each of you states:

- *what* specific things you will do (e.g.; make a note in the patient's chart)

- *when* you will do this (e.g.; within 2 days after I complete an initial evaluation)

- *under what conditions* (e.g.; for each patient with a diagnosis of aphasia to whom I am assigned by my supervisor)

4. Contract period

Because you will be trying to achieve only a limited amount of improvement, the contract period usually should be quite short. Try to limit it to a maximum of two or three weeks. Write down when you agree to start work on the activities you plan and when you will stop to evaluate your success.

5. Plan for monitoring progress

Even though you wait to evaluate your overall success until the end of the contract period, there are several reasons why you should plan some system for keeping track of whether key activities are completed along the way. Doing this can:

- provide encouragement to both of you if things are going well

- let you revise the plan and avoid unnecessary frustration if unexpected obstacles appear early in the contract period

- provide you with a record of what went wrong if either of you occasionally fails to complete your part of the bargain. This information may be helpful when you negotiate your next contract.

Sometimes a 'log' or diary kept by the student is helpful. However, be sure the system you use is not too time consuming or complicated.

6. Rewards and penalties

Since this is your first attempt at a contract, you probably will want to agree on some specific reward the student can earn by keeping her part of the agreement. This may be something the supervisor provides, or simply some privilege the student allows herself. If the student feels she needs it for motivation you also can agree on some modest penalty she will pay in the event she fails. Whatever you plan, try to keep it simple; and, if at all possible, try to think of rewards and penalties that have some logical connection with the behavior about which you are concerned. Remember, eventually the correct behavior needs to be rewarding enough in and of itself for the student to comply consistently on her own. Over-reliance on artificial, extrinsic rewards could make this independent compliance difficult to achieve.

7. Signatures

When you feel your contract is ready to put into action, sign your names to the planning form to show your formal commitment to it. In a real contracting procedure, at this stage you would want to make a copy of the written agreement for each of you to keep.

TASK D **Think briefly about follow-up activities**

The performance problems described at the start of this exercise probably cannot be corrected in a single attempt. Take a few minutes to compare the short-term goal for your contract with your long-range purpose. What remains to be done? See if you can think of a couple of successive goals or types of activities that you might use as the basis for future work on the problem. You don't need to work these out in detail, simply talk briefly about how the process and focus of your contracting might need to change as you progress.

You also should take a few minutes to talk about what you might do if the contract you just drafted turned out not to be realistic. Can you think of ways to make the student's obligations easier to meet if this seems necessary?

LEARNING CONTRACT

1. **Long-range purpose** What we hope to achieve eventually is for

_____to learn to:
(student)

2. **Immediate objective.** By the end of this contract _____ will
(student)
have accomplished the following specific things:

3. **Plan of action.** To achieve this objective, each of us agrees to do the following:

_____ will:
(student)

_____ will:
(instructor)

4. **Time period**

We will start working on these activities on _____

We will complete the activities and evaluate our success on _____

5. **Plan for monitoring progress.** We will keep a simple record of what we do by:

6. **Reward and penalty**

If _____ completes his/her part of this agreement he/she will
    (student)   earn the following reward:

If _____ does not complete his/her part of the agreement he/she
    (student)   agrees to do the following as a penalty:

7. **Signatures**

_____   _____

(student)   (instructor)

_____

(date)

FEEDBACK

FEEDBACK ON EXERCISE 12

The best way to evaluate your work on this exercise is to discuss it with your partner and with several other clinical teachers. The following questions can provide a framework for this review.

To evaluate the contract you wrote, discuss it with another pair of clinical teachers. If possible, talk with partners who also have done this exercise, and who chose the same performance problem as you. This will give you feedback on the clarity, completeness and practicality of your plan, and let you see how someone else approached this problem. Begin by simply reading each other's contracts. Then allow time to ask questions about anything that is unclear and to comment on the contract. Consider both the content of the agreement and the way it is worded. The following list of questions may be used as a checklist for this review:

1. *Is the agreement clearly stated?* Can you visualize what will go on when it is put into action? Pay special attention to the *verbs* used to describe the student's activities. They should be action words that describe specific things you could actually see, hear or feel the student do. (For example, it would be better to say, 'The student agrees to keep a record of the time when she arrived at each meeting she attended and when the meeting actually began' than to say, 'The student will try to be more aware of whether she is punctual.') The instructor's activities should be listed with equal concreteness.

2. *Do the terms of the contract seem realistic?* To assess this you will need to know something about the assumptions made by the partners who drafted the contract when they 'set the scene' for their planning.
   Within this framework think about whether:

   • the student and supervisor will have time to do what they have planned

   • this can be done without disrupting things for other people, violating established rules, or being extravagant in use of resources

   • the student is likely to be successful. Is there a risk this contract will simply set her up for failure by committing her or the instructor to something that is too ambitious?

3. *Does the plan seem useful?* If the short-term goal is achieved, will this be a significant step towards correction of the overall problem? Is this initial improvement likely to last once the contract period is over? Does it provide something the student can build on in the future?

If you and your partner are working alone on this exercise, you could try one of the following to get feedback on what you accomplished:

• ask a 'real' student to critique your contract

• ask other clinicians to review it even if they haven't done the exercise themselves

• put your contract aside for a few days and then try to review it yourselves from a fresh point of view.

To evaluate the process you used to negotiate the contract, discuss it with your partner in the exercise. Consider the following questions:

1. *What sort of working relationship did you establish with your partner?*

The contracting process usually works best if it encourages the student to take initiative and responsibility for finding a way to make improvements in his/her own performance. This sort of climate can be established in many different ways. Both verbal and non-verbal communication are important. For example:

- How was the idea of making a contract presented? Did the instructor's words and tone of voice make it sound like something the student was required to do—or like a suggestion they would explore together?

- Who went first most of the time in proposing ideas for different parts of the contract?

- Did you feel you were really listening to each other? Giving each other time to think and express your ideas without interrupting?

- Who held on to the contract form most of the time? Who did most of the writing?

Talk to your partner about how you felt during the negotiations. What helped you feel free, stimulated your thinking, encouraged you to think of this as your contract? Did your partner do anything that interfered, made you feel intimidated or ignored?

Good beginnings often are especially important. See if you can think of anything the instructor did early in the negotiations to affirm that this was a joint venture, not simply a new way for the teacher to tell the student what to do.

2. How did you handle differences of opinion if they occurred?

This is another important way in which the mutuality of the process is established and maintained. At some point in the planning process one of you is likely to be attracted to an approach the other mistrusts. Sometimes the student may be eager to try something the instructor fears would be too ambitious or difficult to arrange. Or, the instructor may be enthusiastic about an activity the student feels would be boring, intimidating, or simply 'not her style'. If such disagreement arose during your negotiations you should have:

- discussed your feelings openly and honestly

- allowed the student's preferences to prevail most of the time unless this seemed likely to create serious practical problems

- yet tried to make some compromises that let both the instructor's and student's preference be considered and to affirm this as a shared planning process with healthy give and take on both sides.

3. Did you consider alternatives before settling on an agreement?

Even if the first idea one of you suggests looks good to both of you, in the long run the contracting process is most likely to work well if you make a serious attempt to think of several possible ways in which each part of the contract could be designed. This is especially true when the contract being discussed is only the first in a series of plans that will be needed to achieve a long-range change, and when instructor and student are still relative novices in using the technique. The few extra minutes you take to talk about different ways in which you might begin work on the problem can help you:

- get used to exchanging ideas in a relaxed, constructive way

- recognize that the performance problem probably has several different aspects and that full correction is likely to call for a series of different learning plans

- develop ideas for things you can substitute if your initial plan turns out to be unworkable

- make a start on plans for more demanding activities that could be the basis for future contracts if the initial contract goes well.

4. Did you try to predict the practical demands of each alternative?

Before you agree on a plan of action each of you needs to ask yourself how difficult it will be to keep your side of the proposed bargain. To be realistic about your commitments you will need to spell out a list of the specific tasks you will perform and the resources this will require. Usually you should avoid things that are complicated, artificial, or will require other people to change their usual pattern of activity. Give particular attention to discussing whether each of you really will have the time to do all the things you are considering, and whether appropriate opportunities for attempted action will be available when the student needs them.

5. Was the overall tone of your discussion positive?

You do need to be sure you both have a similar view of what the performance problem involves, and discussing a few specific examples of things the student does wrong can be a useful starting point for planning correction. However, the negotiating session should not be used primarily for the instructor to point out to the student in great detail all the flaws in her performance, or for exasperated statements such as, 'I really don't see why this is so hard for you.' The partner who took the part of the instructor in this exercise should have tried in some way to mention and affirm some of the things the student does well, and to encourage the student to select a contract activity that builds on existing strengths and interests. This is more likely to lead to early success and encourage further work on the problem than if the student is made to feel she must tackle the worst part of her performance first.

Planning ahead

Planning for follow-up activities was only a small part of this lengthy exercise, but the following general suggestions may help you in future efforts to decide what to do if things go wrong, and what to do next if the initial contract is a success.

Even a carefully planned contract may be difficult to fulfill. The same factors that created the performance problem in the first place may discourage even modest attempts at change. Unexpected obstacles can interfere with completion of even the simplest activities. When this happens you need to keep an initial failure from being so discouraging to either student or instructor that you abandon the whole project or approach future negotiations with a sense of defeat. Some of the things you can do to make early failure less damaging are:

- Avoid making the penalties for early failure too severe.

- Make sure the system you set up for monitoring completion of agreed activities includes recording of exactly what went wrong if each of you is unable to do all you promised. Reviewing these notes can help you decide whether to respond to initial failure by simply trying again with the original plan or by redesigning the contract to make it less ambitious or to avoid specific obstacles.

- As you discuss what happened be sure to affirm what was accomplished even if you must admit some key activities were not completed.

- Try to shift to constructive planning for another attempt as soon as possible. This will be easiest if your original planning included discussion of alternatives or modifications that could serve as a fall-back approach.

Deciding how to progress from success to success also presents challenges. One of the obvious risks in offering the student an attractive reward for successful completion of specific activities is that once the instructor stops providing this incentive the student's performance will deteriorate. A planned progression in the type and timing of rewards can help to wean the student from dependency on the instructor and make future compliance natural and self-sustaining.

In order to encourage early progress in your initial contract you were advised in the exercise to agree on some immediate, tangible reward. Often this means something the instructor will arrange: time off, an opportunity for the student to do something she particularly enjoys, or special praise. This can be acceptable at first, but in subsequent contracts the rewards should shift:

- away from artificial, extrinsic rewards arranged by the instructor to satisfactions that are a natural consequence of the desired performance itself

- away from immediate, frequent, regular rewards for fairly limited achievement to rewards that are infrequent, sometimes unpredictable or delayed, and received only when compliance is good.

When the positive consequences of independent compliance are likely to be delayed or difficult to perceive, contracting may need to help the student learn to find satisfaction simply in knowing she is able to stick to a pattern of behavior she knows intellectually is good. This means finding ways to help the student reshape her own self image to see herself as a 'winner' capable of controlling her own actions rather than a 'loser' who lacks the will-power to do what she knows is best. In her exceptional book on methods for helping students overcome persistent problems in basic writing skills, Mina Shaughnessy captured the essence of this sort of growth towards student self-motivation when she wrote:

This discovery by a student that he can do something he thought he couldn't releases the energy to do it. Students who make many errors feel helpless about correcting them. Error has them in its power, forcing them to hide or bluff or feign indifference, but never to attack. The teacher must encourage an aggressive attitude toward error and then provide a strategy for its defeat, one that allows the student to count his victories as he goes and thereby grow in confidence. This means letting the student in on what is happening—setting a reasonable limit to what he needs to accomplish (the reduction of errors per 300 words from 15 to 6 in one semester, for example), helping him classify the kinds of errors he makes most often (the discovery that although he has 20 errors he has only 5 problems is in itself encouraging to a student), and then planning instruction so that success is built into each lesson and the student can see that he is finally beginning to cope with errors.[4]

If we can accomplish this the student will have the emotional energy needed to progress to self-contracting, and will be well on the way to replacing an unwanted old habit with a new pattern of independent success.

Of course all this takes time. Both student and instructor must be prepared to invest considerable wit and energy in order to use contracting as a tool for improving motivation and compliance. However, one has only to compare this with the immense amounts of time and effort that can be squandered on coping with the results of habitually flawed performance to realize contracting can be a good investment.

GIVING STUDENTS A SENSE OF POWER

In his book *The Psychology of Hope*[5] Ezra Stotland discusses three closely related emotions:

- *Hope*— a feeling of confidence that good things will occur; an expectation that good things can be achieved
- *Motivation*— willingness to attempt to achieve a goal
- *Persistence*— willingness to try repeatedly in spite of initial failure or lack of knowledge of the results of earlier action.

These feelings are incorporated in the concept described so clearly by Judith Miller and her colleagues;[6]

- *Power* — an individual's expectation that his own actions can influence his well-being, his feeling that he has some degree of control over his environment and over what other people do to and for him.

These feelings are of particular importance when patients, staff or students are expected to learn things that are unpleasant, uncertain or difficult. Such challenges are common in clinical teaching. The average health professional's job includes a variety of tasks that are frustrating, boring, frightening, uncomfortable or unpleasant. Patients too must learn to carry out activities that are embarrassing, tedious or unappealing. Using a wheelchair in public, giving up favorite foods or prized activities, taking care of an osteotomy or applying medication to a skin disorder are all examples of actions that demand emotional sturdiness of the performer. Teaching our students *how* to do such things is not enough. We also must help them develop the sense of power that reassures them these punishing efforts will be worthwhile.

The student's willingness to assume responsibility depends on his belief that he is capable of acting effectively. This feeling of power is strongly influenced by the climate of expectations and relationships in which the technical side of instruction takes place. The final section of this chapter focuses, therefore, not on the mechanics of a special teaching method, but on something more basic—the infrastructure of small, commonplace actions with which our formal instruction is surrounded. These unplanned, and often unexamined, actions can have a powerful effect on the student's sense of personal hope and power.

Unfortunately, many of our first contacts with students in the clinic seem designed to reduce their initiative and sense of control. In its early stages clinical teaching often is highly informational and authoritarian. The timing, purpose, content and format of instruction are usually established unilaterally by the teacher, and efforts to develop the student's independent initiative set aside until he has 'gotten the basics'. Certainly one can make a strong argument for letting the experts do most of the initial instructional planning. The new patient, novice staff member and beginning student often have little idea what they need to learn and even less idea how to go about learning it. Yet eventually these students must learn to make persistent, independent, correct use of the information and skills the expert teaches them. This will be difficult to accomplish if they have inadvertently been made to feel dependent and powerless.

The following exercise will let you practice identifying examples of simple 'background' events that might reduce a patient's sense of power and ask you to think of ways in which the clinical teacher could provide necessary technical instruction within a framework that encourages the learner to take control.

POWER SHARING—MAKING THE LITTLE THINGS ADD UP

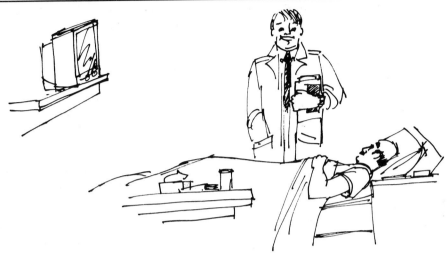

You can do this exercise entirely on your own, or do the initial tasks alone and then discuss your ideas with other teachers who have analyzed the same case. Whichever you do, please remember your concern in this exercise should *not* be with the technical merits of the teaching materials used or the content covered by the teacher in the case. Please focus your attention on all of the little things this teacher does (or fails to do) as he interacts with the patient he is teaching. Think about the type of relationship this establishes and how it may influence the patient's sense of responsibility and control over his own well-being.

TASK A

Begin by reading quickly through the attached case description to get a general idea of what happens.

TASK B

Next, go back over the case carefully and *underline* each part of the narrative or dialogue that you feel represents an action that could affect the patient's feelings of power. Look both for points at which you think the teacher did something or failed to do something you think is important.

TASK C

In the margin of the case description:

- put a + symbol next to anything you think would enhance the patient's sense of power
- put a – symbol next to anything you think might make this patient feel powerless.

TASK D

Select any two points at which you marked the teacher's actions with a – symbol. For each of these try to think of one concrete thing you believe the instructor could have done instead *or* added to his performance to help the patient feel greater control. Make notes of your ideas. Be as specific as possible. Remember, in this exercise it's the 'little things' we're interested in.

TASK E

If you have arranged to exchange ideas with other teachers, do so now by comparing your scoring of events in the case and your suggestions for practical ways to give the patient power. Then turn to the feedback section.

CASE DESCRIPTION

Arnold Polinsky is a 58-year-old taxi driver who entered the hospital 4 days ago for removal of a rectal tumor. He tolerated surgery well and has been fitted with a colostomy bag. David Burke, a staff nurse specializing in osteotomy care, has been asked to start teaching him the self-care procedures he will need to follow when he goes home.

David arrived at Mr Polinsky's semi-private room at about 4 p.m. and found him in bed, watching the baseball game on television. The elderly patient in the next bed was asleep and snoring steadily. David entered the room, walked to the end of the bed, and said, 'Hi, Mr Polinsky. I'm David Burke. Your surgeon asked me to come show you what you're going to have to do to look after that bag he fitted you with the other day after your surgery.' 'Oh, hi doctor', replied Mr Polinsky. 'Sorry,' replied David, smiling, 'I should have explained. I'm not a doctor. I'm the Osteotomy Nurse Specialist.' 'Oh, excuse me.' 'That's okay', David responded, walking over to the television. 'Now, let's just switch this off so you can hear, okay?' 'Say,' David continued, 'aren't you supposed to be out of bed now?' 'I just got back in a couple of minutes before you came', Mr Polinsky explained apologetically. 'I was up most of the afternoon and I got kinda pooped.' 'Okay,' said David, 'now, let me just crank your bed up a little more so you can see better. I've brought some things I think will help you see how this bag works and what you need to do to look after it.' David opened a kit of materials used for this teaching and began his explanation.

Fifteen minutes later, after going over the basic procedure for removing and attaching the bag and for cleaning the stoma, David reassured Mr Polinsky, 'This really won't seem so hard once you've tried it a couple of times.' Then he looked at his watch and continued, 'I think that's enough for one day. I've still got to see another patient on this floor before the supper trays come up.' He then pulled out a booklet, and handed it to Mr Polinsky, saying, 'Here's something that explains most of the things we've just gone over. I'd like you to have a look at it tonight to go over them again.' As he turned to leave, David added, 'If you watch really closely when the nurse comes to change your bag tonight, you'll see how quick and easy it is once you've learned how. So long, Mr Polinsky. See you tomorrow.' 'So long', replied the patient.

EXERCISE 13

FEEDBACK

FEEDBACK ON EXERCISE 13

Perhaps the easiest method for analyzing the many different ways in which a teacher's interaction with a student can influence the student's self-confidence and sense of power is to think in terms of several broad categories of action. These include actions that increase or diminish the student's feelings of:

- *Environmental control*

The patient in his hospital bed, like the student or staff member beginning work in a new department, finds himself in an unfamiliar environment. The well-known sights and smells of home are missing, telephone and eyeglasses often frustratingly out of reach, and other people determine even such simple things as whether the lights are on or off and the door open or shut. Even when their actions are 'standard procedure' and represent attempts to keep the patient safe, staff routines often continuously erode the patient's sense of control. In this case, for example, David entered the patient's room without knocking, turned off the television and cranked up the bed with only a token explanation or 'OK?', and left the room without any effort to discover whether the patient wanted to return to watching the ball game or wanted anything else that was out of easy reach, adjusted or brought closer. Such simple actions take little time, but do help to establish that this is the patient's territory and that he should be allowed a reasonable degree of control over it. Several points at which David seemed to deprive Mr Polinsky of environmental control are marked on the feedback sheet at the end of the comments with the symbol − E.

- *Uncertainty*

The health care process involves a steady stream of mysterious events for most patients. Objects and terms that seem commonplace to the professionals who use them many times each day may be confusing and even threatening to the layman. The identity of the many people who come and go uninvited in his room is often unclear, and the schedule for what will happen next may seem like a closely guarded secret to the patient.

In this case the nurse-instructor did several simple, but useful, things to reduce this uncertainty. He began by telling the patient his name and explaining why he was there. He made at least a brief attempt to explain why he was doing such things as turning off the television and cranking up the bed, and he gave Mr Polinsky a booklet that allowed him to study in writing terms and diagrams that may have been difficult to grasp when they were explained initially. However, the patient was clearly unsure exactly who David was, may have been put on the defensive by being corrected, and perhaps had little idea what an 'osteotomy nurse specialist' was even after this title was announced. David also ended his session with Mr. Polinsky on a note of mystery—telling him 'I'll see you tomorrow', without even a hint as to whether he could be expected to return at the same time as today or at some different point in the patient's highly unpredictable (at least to him) day. All these are little things, but they do add up. Even if he is given no control over who comes and goes and when, Mr Polinsky probably will feel less at sea if he at least knows what to expect.

In the feedback script several events that seem likely to add to the patient's uncertainty are marked −U, and several that prevent or reduce uncertainty are marked +U. You may have thought of others that could have the same types of effect.

● *Independence and individual identity*

Influential actions in this category include all the many things the instructor does to affirm or negate that he sees the patient as a mature, responsible person with his own individual interests, talents and life-history. Unfortunately, in this case the instructor did little or nothing to show he recognized Mr Polinsky as a real person. David did greet the patient by name, but apart from that seemed to regard him as simply another in a chain of interchangeable patients with ostomies. His manner was not unfriendly, simply very impersonal. This was compounded by his making it clear that he was also in something of a hurry to get on to his next patient. By the time he is discharged, Mr Polinsky will need to take the initiative in carrying out the procedures he has learned for managing his ostomy. He must do this correctly and conscientiously, and may find he has to adapt his usual life-style in order to accommodate these new responsibilities. David could begin now to foster the sense of personal power such compliance will require by showing from the start that he thinks of his patient as another valued adult. Even so simple an act as taking a moment to chat with Mr Polinsky about whether he is a baseball fan could begin to put their relationship on this basis.

David did do several useful things that should have implied to Mr Polinsky that he was being thought of as someone who is capable of learning to care for his ostomy and who will be expected to do so. Charles Cooley summarized the influence a teacher's expectations can have when he wrote:

In the presence of one whom we feel to be of importance there is a tendency to enter into and adopt, by sympathy, his judgment of ourselves, to put a new value on ideas and purposes, to recast life in his image . . . our personality grows and takes form by divining the appearance of our present self to other minds.[7]

By giving his patient a booklet and saying, 'I'd like you to have a look at it tonight' and by asking Mr Polinsky to watch closely when the nurse changed his ostomy bag, David was doing much more than simply directing his student to useful sources of information. He was also establishing an expectation that Mr Polinsky would follow through on his own.

David was less constructive in the way he handled the question of Mr Polinsky being in bed when he arrived. Although his question showed he expected the patient to follow through conscientiously on the staff recommendation that he get up as much as possible, his approach seemed to put Mr Polinsky on the defensive. David also did nothing to reinforce the patient's good compliance when it was reported. This whole exchange could have been more positive if David had rephrased his question to ask something such as, 'How are you doing with staying up and out of bed today?' and had responded to Mr Polinsky's report with slightly more enthusiasm.

These efforts to give the patient a greater sense of control could be extended by adding a few simple opportunities for him to make active choices about the structure of his instruction. There may be relatively little opportunity for flexibility in key aspects of the procedure for ostomy care itself; however David could let the patient make decisions about how he would prefer to learn these. For example, he could ask the patient whether he would like to examine the sample materials or just have David explain them. Would he like the door to the room open or closed when David leaves? Does he have any preference for when the next lesson is scheduled? David probably already has a number of appointments scheduled for the next day, so he can't simply ask, 'When would you like me to come?' He could say, however, 'I'm free tomorrow at—and at—. Would one of those times be better for you than the other?' To let the patient help determine the focus of future lessons, David might suggest Mr Polinsky keep a list of any questions he has as he reads the booklet and watches the nurse so they can discuss these tomorrow.

Some of the positive and negative actions related to the patient's independence and identity are marked in the margin of the case with a +I or –I. Several points at which additional actions might have been useful are marked with an add I.

The specific actions discussed in this case all seem quite unimportant if they are considered one at a time. Taken collectively, however, they add up to a powerful tool for building or destroying the attitudinal foundation for future compliance. As you complete this exercise, take a few minutes to think about the many parallels between the patient in this case and the novice student or staff member. Such special techniques for improving compliance as values analysis and contracting may depend for their effectiveness on our skill in using small actions to share power with the people we teach.

CASE DESCRIPTION

Arnold Polinsky is a 58-year-old taxi driver who entered the hospital 4 days ago for removal of a rectal tumour. He tolerated surgery well and has been fitted with a colostomy bag. David Burke, a staff nurse specializing in osteotomy care, has been asked to start teaching him the self-care procedures he will need to follow when he goes home.

David arrived at Mr Polinsky's semi-private room at about 4 p.m. and found him in bed, watching the baseball game on television. The elderly patient in the next bed was asleep and snoring steadily. David entered the room, walked to the end of the bed, and said, 'Hi, Mr Polinsky. I'm David Burke. Your surgeon asked me to come show you what you're going to have to do to look after that bag he fitted you with the other day after your surgery.' 'Oh, hi doctor', replied Mr Polinsky. 'Sorry,' replied David, smiling, 'I should have explained. I'm not a doctor. I'm the osteotomy nurse specialist.' 'Oh, excuse me.' 'That's okay', David responded, walking over to the television. 'Now, let's just switch this off so you can hear, okay?' 'Say,' David continued, 'aren't you supposed to be out of bed now?' 'I just got back in a couple of minutes before you came', Mr Polinsky explained apologetically. 'I was up most of the afternoon and I got kinda pooped.' 'Okay,' said David, 'now, let me just crank your bed up a little more so you can see better. I've brought some things I think will help you see how this bag works and what you need to do to look after it.' David opened a kit of materials used for this teaching and began his explanation.

Fifteen minutes later, after going over the basic procedure for removing and attaching the bag and for cleaning the stoma, David reassured Mr Polinsky, 'This really won't seem so hard once you've tried it a couple of times.' Then he looked at his watch and continued, 'I think that's enough for one day. I've still got to see another patient on this floor before the supper trays come up.' He then pulled out a booklet, and handed it to Mr Polinsky, saying, 'Here's something that explains most of the things we've just gone over. I'd like you to have a look at it tonight to go over them again.' As he turned to leave, David added, 'If you watch really closely when the nurse comes to change your bag tonight, you'll see how quick and easy it is once you've learned how. So long, Mr Polinsky. See you tomorrow.' 'So long', replied the patient.

NOTES TO CHAPTER 3

1. Rosenstock I M 1966 Why people use health services. Milbank Memorial Fund Quarterly 44: 94–127. Becker M H 1974 The health belief model and sick role behavior. Health Education Monograph 2: 409–419
2. Belloc N B, Breslow 1972 The relation of physical health status and health practices. Preventive Medicine 1: 409–21. Belloc, Breslow 1973 Relationship of health practices and mortality. Preventive Medicine 2: 67–81
3. Lewin K 1951 Field theory in social science. New York, Harper
4. Shaughnessy M 1977 Errors and expectations: A guide for the teacher of basic writing. Oxford University Press, New York, pp 125
5. Stotland E 1969 The psychology of hope. Jossey-Bass, San Francisco
6. Miller J (ed) 1983 Coping with chronic illness: overcoming powerlessness. F A David, Philadelphia
7. Cooley C 1922 Human nature and the social order. Charles Scribner, New York, pp 206–207b

4 USING FAMILIAR METHODS OF INSTRUCTION EFFECTIVELY

THE NEED FOR MODIFICATION

Classroom and clinical teachers use many of the same instructional methods. In both settings instructors show, tell, question, model, coach, counsel, correct and direct; but when the clinical teacher does these things the techniques she uses often take on some very special qualities. Lecturing provides a particularly obvious example. As do their colleagues in the classroom, clinical teachers spend much of their time explaining things and giving their students information, directions and advice. Sometimes this 'telling' is done through a conventional lecture: at a scheduled hour, in a classroom or amphitheatre, with a group of seated students listening and taking notes as the instructor speaks. More often, however, the clinical lecture is given:

- to an audience of only one or two
- in a work area or patient's room where many other things may be going on at the same time
- on an apparently impromptu basis as the need arises and the opportunity presents itself.

Throughout the day in most hospitals one can see such 'minilectures' taking place: in the coffee shop, at the elevators, in emergency room cubicles, on stairways and at the nurses' station. Sometimes they have been scheduled in advance, but frequently these lessons are initiated by a question, an error, or by an event the instructor wants to be sure the student notices and understands. Even the conventional lectures given by clinical teachers often have some unusual features. For example, staff in-service lectures often:

- address an audience that includes some staff who know a great deal about the topic and others who know next to nothing
- are presented in response to a very vague request, such as, 'We'd like to hear something new about pain management'
- are isolated, 'one shot' presentations rather than part of a course of organized instruction
- involve little or no advance preparation or formal follow-up study by the people who attend
- are not followed by formal testing to find out whether the listeners have actually learned anything from the experience.

In addition, the timing of attendance may be highly erratic. Because staff must fit the lecture in between a variety of other work activities, some listeners arrive late, others leave early, and there are often a few who seem to pause only long enough to consume the snack they have brought with them before they hurry off to some other assignment. Teaching by telling under such conditions clearly requires major modifications in the lecture techniques used by most classroom teachers. The same is often true of many other familiar instructional methods.

COMMON PROBLEMS IN CLINICAL TEACHING

Several of the most significant special features of the clinical teaching environment were mentioned briefly in the Introduction to this Handbook. Before beginning discussion of specific methods of teaching, we should examine these characteristics in more detail to identify some of the problems they create. Some common disorders of clinical instruction and the factors that help to produce them are:

- *Superficiality*

Opportunities for learning in the clinical setting are so varied and abundant that teachers and students often are tempted to try to do a little of everything. The result can be failure to make a useful amount of progress in any one area. Selectivity is a continual challenge.

● *Fragmentation*

The schedule for many key activities cannot be fully controlled. Sometimes it cannot even be fully predicted by the clinical teacher. Logical progression and grouping of related activities is difficult to arrange. Patients may be taught by professionals from several different fields, and fieldwork students often have clinical supervisors who are not part of their academic faculty. These factors create obstacles to tying together learning, especially when it occurs in bits and pieces over a long period of time.

● *Wastefulness*

Even when the clinical teacher is highly selective, many excellent opportunities for learning are difficult to use efficiently. Some important events occur unexpectedly and are ignored or used poorly because the instructor had not planned for them. Students work without direct supervision much of the time. They may fail to notice important events, and make errors or achieve wonders without this being reinforced by the instructor.

● *Error*

In the classroom the well-prepared teacher is seldom 'wrong'. Academic teaching is supported by logic and the scientific literature. The rules of procedure and supporting theory taught are general and based on statistical averages for large numbers of cases. By contrast, in the clinic authority is continually tested by practical results, and the uncertainty of clinical science makes mistakes inevitable. Many of the things clinical teachers suggest to patients, students and colleagues simply turn out not to work. Unless both student and instructor can deal constructively with the senior clinician's fallibility both may be immobilized by it.

● *Ambiguity*

The student's role is complex and often confusing. Adult patients are expected to follow the advice

of young strangers simply because they are professionals. Students and staff trainees must shift from receiving criticism and directions from their instructors one minute to answering patients' questions with authority the next. As the end of training or the day of discharge approaches, expectations may change abruptly and a person who has been criticized for not following directions obediently one day may be criticized for not showing initiative the next.

The rest of this chapter will be devoted to an examination of a few of the ways in which familiar instructional techniques can be modified to avoid and cope with these problems. Each section will include an exercise in the form of a case problem with accompanying questions. You can complete these exercises alone and use the feedback sections to help you review your work. However, the exercises will be more interesting and valuable if you can arrange to work on them with at least one other clinical teacher. In that case, begin by answering the questions independently. Then exchange ideas with a partner or other members of a small group. Finally, compare what you have done with the comments in the feedback pages. The problems presented by the cases are complex, and might be solved in a variety of ways. Whether you work alone or with others don't hesitate to disagree with or add to the necessarily limited suggestions included in the feedback sections.

This review of familiar instructional methods will begin with the one just discussed—the lecture.

LECTURES

The lecture is a technique for teaching by telling and learning by listening. First and foremost it is a tool for giving students information. However, oral telling has the potential for doing much more than this. It also can be a powerful tool for stimulating thought, for provoking students to respond and react to the information they receive.

Whether a lecture is given briefly, on the run, to a single student; or for an hour to a seated audience of 60, to use the technique effectively the lecturer must grapple with a series of demanding questions.

1. What information do the listeners really need? How can I avoid wasting their time and mine

telling them things:
- they already know
- they probably will never use, or that
- they could get more efficiently from a book, a handout or a self-instructional unit?

2. What can I do to stimulate active listening? How do I expect the listeners will use the information I present and what can I say to encourage them to practice that sort of use as I lecture?

3. How can I present my material so it is interesting, easy to understand and easy to remember?

4. How can I keep the listener's attention from wandering? What can I do to reduce such practical obstacles to attention as fatigue, boredom, confusion and preoccupation with other concerns?

The following case illustrates the practical challenges answering these questions often presents when lecturing is done in a clinical setting.

EXERCISE 14

GIVING INFORMATION, DIRECTIONS AND ADVICE: THE CASE OF THE DISCOURAGED LECTURER

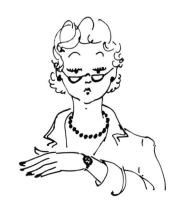

Ethel Andersen is Director of the Department of Speech-Language Pathology at a 225-bed rehabilitation hospital. Several weeks ago she was asked to give a 40 minute orientation lecture to newly hired staff nurses as part of their orientation to the hospital. Miss Andersen had done this before; in fact, she has been asked to present orientation lectures for nursing and several other departments at least twice a year for the past several years. She was told to expect about 10 nurses for this lecture.

Because she usually includes a brief tour of the department as part of this type of class, Miss Andersen scheduled the lecture in the department at 1 o'clock in the afternoon when her department is usually not too busy. She began promptly at the scheduled time, even though only five nurses had arrived. She explained they needed to get started because there was a lot to cover. Three more new staff arrived one at a time during the first 10 minutes of her presentation.

Miss Andersen began with the topic she felt was most important, a summary of the different services her department provides. This took about 5 minutes. She then went on to tell the group:

- how many staff work in the department and what their qualifications are
- a little about the history of the department
- how patients are referred for service
- how many patients the department has served in the last 3 years
- how the pattern of problems referred has changed since the department was started
- what hours the department is open
- what some of their current problems are.

As she began explaining that the department is currently very short of staff and has a long waiting list for some types of treatment, Miss Andersen noticed that two people in the back of the room were leaving. She looked at her watch, realized she had run 5 minutes over the allotted time, apologized, and said she was sorry but they would have to tour the department some other day. She asked if there were any questions. There were none. She dismissed the group.

Two days later Miss Andersen ran into the Director of Nursing in the staff cafeteria. The Nursing Director thanked her for the class, and said that turnover had been so great that they would be getting another group for orientation soon. She added, however, that she wasn't sure they'd have time for the 'usual orientation lecture' because things on the units were 'pretty hectic right now'. She asked Miss Andersen whether she thought that would be all right. Miss Andersen responded, 'Whatever you want is okay with me.' The Nursing Director replied that they'd probably pass up the lecture this time. Miss Andersen felt a little crestfallen, but made no comment.

She returned to her office after lunch and told her assistant what had happened, saying, 'That's fine with me. I've got plenty of other work to do.' Her assistant replied, 'You sure do! Besides, the new nurses in this place are really hopeless. It always takes a couple of months and lots of yelling from us before they fill out the referral forms correctly and send them down on time . . . .'

and they never do seem to understand that we can't schedule patients on Thursday morning when we have our special clinic going on.' Think about your own answers to the following two questions, and try to discuss them with at least one other clinical teacher before you turn to the feedback section.

1. If you were Miss Andersen, would you agree the orientation lecture should be cancelled?
2. If you were asked to give this lecture, would you do anything differently? Why?

FEEDBACK ON EXERCISE 14

Would you agree that the future orientation lectures should be cancelled? This certainly is tempting; but is it wise? The staff member's comments in the last paragraph of the case suggest that orientation of new nurses may, in fact, be needed. However, the case tells you nothing about what Miss Andersen or the Director of Nursing hoped this class would accomplish. To decide whether future lectures would be worthwhile you would need to begin by spelling out exactly what useful things they could help the new nurses learn. Then you must judge whether this learning would be likely to improve their efficiency, effectiveness or morale sufficiently to make the class worth the time and effort it will cost.

Whatever you decide about the overall value of an orientation class, simply repeating the sort of lecture described in the case seems unwise. Some of the problems and potential changes you might have identified include:

1. Much of the content presented was probably irrelevant so far as the nurses' future responsibilities are concerned. A smattering of departmental history and recitation of referral statistics seem unlikely to help the nurses much in their future contacts with the speech-language department. Some of the other topics Miss Andersen covered do seem potentially useful, but their importance is difficult to judge without some analysis of the tasks the nurses will be assigned and of their current level of knowledge about speech therapy. You might have proposed gathering information to help you plan this lecture by:

- Asking your own staff what they think the nurses need to know

- Talking to several more experienced nurses to see what they found confusing in their early contacts with your department

- Taking a few minutes at the start of the lecture to ask the new staff what previous contacts they have had with a speech therapy department, and whether they have any questions they would like you to answer

- Reviewing your own experience to think of problems that have occurred frequently in the past or to identify new ways in which your department and nursing could work together more productively.

These methods provide less detailed information than the full process of learning needs assessment described in Chapter 2 of this Handbook; but even such a brief review can help you set reasonable objectives and select relevant content for this lecture.

2. The lecture was a very passive experience for the staff who attended, and many probably found their attention wandering. The topics covered in a lecture such as this not only need to be relevant, they should *seem* useful to the listeners. One of the great advantages the clinical teacher enjoys is the immediacy with which students can apply the information they are given. This application is especially helpful if it is used as a framework for the lecture, and if 'telling' by the teacher is combined with frequent 'doing' by the students. You might have proposed a variety of techniques for making this lecture more practical and interactive. The approach you select will depend a great deal on the objectives you establish. Here are a few examples:

- If one of your objectives is for the nurses to learn how to fill out referral forms correctly, instead of simply describing the correct procedure you could give each nurse a copy of the form, provide a brief summary of information on a patient for whom referral would be appropriate, and ask each person to fill out the form for the patient. By providing feedback with a correctly completed form on an overhead transparency you could stress some of the points that are likely to be confusing and connect your comments to the work the class has just done instead of talking in the abstract.

- If one of your objectives is for the nurses to remember what types of services your department provides and to recognize which of their patients might benefit from referral, you might begin this part of the lecture by giving the class brief descriptions of several patients, some good candidates for referral, others not. The nurses could then be asked to review these cases during a lecture on general guidelines for referral, and then to decide which patients they expect would benefit from your services. A short group discussion of their responses would let you recognize and reinforce correct applications of your guidelines and clarify or repeat any points that were overlooked or misinterpreted.

3. This was an inefficient method of distributing standardized information. The new nurses probably do need to know such things as the hours the department is open, the names of staff, and the telephone number to call if they have questions. However, such facts are easily forgotten and can be provided just as well on a written handout or by putting them in the procedure manual on the nursing units. This would let you save time during the lecture for more interactive instruction and for presenting information that requires interpretation.

4. The timing and location of the lecture seem poor. As a clinical teacher you often have more choice in deciding where and when a lecture will take place than does the average classroom instructor. In this case, however, Miss Andersen seems to have made a number of poor decisions. Problems and potential solutions you might have thought of include:

- The many late arrivals suggest this class was scheduled at a time when the staff had conflicting assignments. You would be wise to check on the students' schedules first, instead of arbitrarily arranging this lecture at a time that was good for you.

- The lecture was given soon after the nurses were employed and may have come before they had a clear picture of what their specific duties and case load would be. Crowding all orientation activities into their employees' first few days on the job may make the classes easy to schedule; but this makes it difficult to explain how the information you present can be applied, and seems sure to create 'information overload' and confusion. Some other parts of nurses' orientation may need to be immediate, but you would probably find this lecture more beneficial if it were delayed until the new staff feel at home in their jobs.

- The lecture was given in the department so it could end with a brief tour of the department. However, it was planned for a time when the department was not busy and the tour was dropped because the lecturer ran out of time. Holding the class in a place where seating and acoustics were probably not ideal seems foolish unless you take advantage of the location to let the students see things that are difficult to describe in words. In many departments this means letting the students see people and activities, not just empty rooms and unused equipment. However, bringing in a group of outsiders may be disruptive when treatment is in progress. If you feel a tour of some sort is needed, you may want to approach it quite differently. For example, instead of trying to incorporate this in a group lecture, you might suggest to the Director of Nursing that sometime after the first few weeks on the job each new nurse be permitted to leave her unit for half an hour in order to accompany a patient from the floor to speech therapy. If the nurses were given routine information about department services and forms in writing, and the speech therapist's treatment objectives were available to the nurse before her visit began, a 30 minute period of observation and discussion with the therapist and patient might entirely replace the group lecture. This is one of the many situations in which clinical staff can provide needed explanations through 'minilectures' timed to coincide with thought-provoking practical events. The lecture then becomes a timely two-way conversation instead of a detached monologue, and the information exchanged is likely to be memorable and clear.

- If future orientation classes are to involve any sort of group instruction, you will need to plan more carefully for how to deal with late arrivals. In a clinical setting, even if classes are scheduled at times most convenient for the staff, some people still may be delayed by unexpected problems. By starting her lecture with the topic she considered most important, even though half the expected class had not yet arrived, Miss Andersen clearly defeated her own purpose. The beginning and end of the classes are often the times when students are most distracted. Prime time for the topics with highest priority usually comes nearer the middle of the session. If the class begins with a presentation of an organizing outline or problem, this can be distributed in writing or put on the blackboard for students to see if they arrive late. This can make it possible for the late arrivals to catch up without disrupting the class. At other times a sentence or two of explanation from the instructor can help latecomers understand what is taking place and keep them from feeling completely at sea during the rest of the class.

You might have proposed many different ways in which this lecture could be improved. The methods singled out for attention in these comments were selected because they reflect several elements that are important not just in this case, but whenever the lecture method is used. These include:

— clear objectives for the class based on

— a practical assessment of student needs and responsibilities,

— selective presentation of content,

— use of written materials to replace or supplement oral presentation of standardized information,

— use of interactive methods or a questioning/problem-solving framework that allows students to organize the information they receive along practical lines and to apply it without delay, and

— sensible scheduling to avoid practical obstacles to communication and give students information at a time when they are ready to absorb and use it.

DEMONSTRATIONS

Demonstrations are used most frequently for teaching skills that involve movement or interaction when it is easier to show than to tell the student what to do. However, effective demonstrations usually involve more than simply 'showing' by the instructor. The model performance is ordinarily followed by a 'return demonstration' by the student in which he attempts to duplicate the performance he has seen. This process could be called 'learning by imitation'. For teaching by demonstration to be successful the student must first acquire a clear vision of how the procedure is to be carried out, and then become able to execute with his own body the steps he sees in his 'mind's eye'.

The student probably goes through several quite different stages in mastering such an imitation, moving from:

- initial acquisition of a cognitive picture of the procedure by conceptualizing performance as a list of verbal cues,
  to
- development of a 'perceptual blueprint' of performance, a blueprint composed at first of visual images of someone else's actions, but later relying heavily on proprioceptive or emotional cues generated by his own performance and the reaction of others.

Research on motor learning provides fascinating insights into how manipulation of verbal and sensory input, and variations in the pattern of active practice by the student, may influence learning of a new motor skill. The combined effect of these factors is clearly complex, and too dependent upon the characteristics of the skill being learned for us to generate a single list of specific characteristics needed in all good demonstrations. However, this research does show us that to make effective use of demonstrations we must consider the process of learning by imitation as a whole. We must consider not only what we will show the student and how, but how we will back this up with verbal intructions, and how we can arrange for the student to experience a correct performance for himself.

As you review the case in Exercise 15, try to judge both the adequacy of the verbal, visual and practice components of instruction and the logic with which these elements are related to one another.

SHOWING STUDENTS WHAT TO DO: THE CASE OF THE DETERMINED DEMONSTRATOR

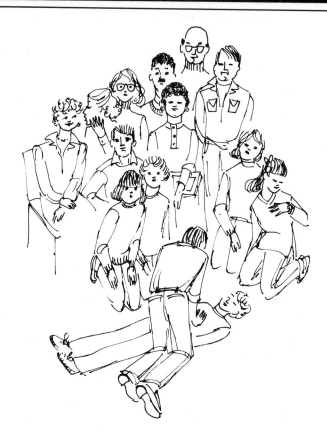

Arthur Wolfe is a pharmacist employed in a recently-opened community health center which provides out-patient services for an inner city neighborhood. Three years ago he enrolled in an evening course on cardiopulmonary resuscitation (CPR) given by the Heart Association. He felt the course was valuable, and enrolled in subsequent courses on advanced life support techniques and training for CPR instructors. He is now one of two certified CPR instructors employed by the health center. As part of its community outreach program, the center began last year to offer free lectures and workshops for laymen in the neighborhood on various health topics. This week, for the first time, the center is offering a basic CPR course as part of this community series. It is being taught in the Center's main waiting room in the early evening after the usual clinic hours. Instruction is divided into three 2-hour classes held on Monday, Wednesday and Friday evenings.

During the first class the first hour was spent showing the students a film which explained the basic anatomy and physiology underlying CPR, showed someone doing one-man and two-man CPR on a mannikin, and demonstrated the procedure for helping someone with an obstructed airway. The film ended with an episode in which a man is shown having a cardiac arrest and being resuscitated by a properly trained layman. Following the film Arthur, who is serving as chief instructor for the course, gave a brief lecture reviewing the main points in CPR procedure, discussing some of the legal questions of greatest concern in doing CPR, and presenting Heart

Association guidelines for health habits that can help prevent heart disease. Each member of the class was then given an instructional booklet summarizing the information covered in the lecture and film, and presenting step-by-step instructions for performing the procedures. These suggested key words to use for recalling each step and were illustrated with clear drawings and diagrams.

The second hour was scheduled for 'hands on' practice by the class. Because there were 23 people enrolled, the class was divided into two groups, each with its own instructor. Loretta Morris, the second instructor, took half the class to another room. Arthur had 12 in his group. During the hour:

— He began by briefly describing the basic steps in the one and two-man CPR procedures (this took about 5 minutes).

— Then he showed the group the practice mannikins (a standard adult model with a gauge attached to show pressure from chest compression, and a baby model) and explained how much they cost and why they needed to be used carefully. He also talked briefly about the need to clean the mannikins carefully after each use for mouth-to-mouth breathing practice to prevent spread of colds or other infections (10 minutes).

— Next, Arthur demonstrated the following procedures:

  • one and two-man CPR on the adult mannikin (a class member with some previous training assisted in the two-man procedure)

  • CPR for infants on the baby mannikin

  • The Heimlich maneuver for clearing an airway obstruction
  (using a class member as subject and simulating the abdominal compression without actual pressure)

  These demonstrations were done with the mannikins on the floor in the center of the room (space cleared by pushing chairs aside) and the students standing around watching and taking notes. As he went through each procedure, Arthur verbally described what he was doing and stopped after each step to point out key aspects of the part of the procedure just demonstrated. (Total time for the demonstrations was 30 minutes.)

— Finally, Arthur asked if there were any questions. There were none (1 minute).

He then suggested the students use the remaining time to practice with the mannikins (14 minutes). One student began practicing with the adult mannikin, trying to do chest compressions. After a few minutes three others took turns doing the same thing, while two others took turns handling the baby and trying to do mouth-to-mouth breathing on it. Arthur moved from one group to the other, correcting several errors in hand placement, and praising a class member who quickly succeeded in delivering chest compressions that registered in the correct range on the pressure gauge attached to the adult mannikin. The other students observed.

As the first class broke up, Arthur reassured them that they would all have a chance to practice on Wednesday, and urged them to study their hand-outs before that class.

The class on Wednesday was scheduled primarily as practice time. However, as the first students to arrive began work with the mannikins, Arthur noticed a great many errors and considerable confusion. After 20 minutes he decided the students would benefit from a repeat demonstration of the one and two-man CPR procedures. He called them together in the center of the room and demonstrated these again. As on Monday, Arthur stopped from time to time to point out key features of performance and to remind the class why they were important.

The students then resumed practice, taking turns on the mannikins until all had tried at least one of the two procedures. About half the class were able to do both. Arthur encouraged the people who were waiting for the adult mannikin to try the Heimlich maneuver on a partner—reminding them not to actually do an abdominal compression. All class members also had a chance to work briefly with the baby. Throughout the practice period Arthur moved from group to group giving feedback and encouragement.

By the end of the class five or six of the students appeared to be doing the procedures well. Others, however, still made major errors or appeared very uncertain in their performance. Arthur had not had a chance to observe a few class members in action. He reminded the group that the final class on Friday was to be used primarily for their written test and for individual practical exams. He urged them all to study their handouts in preparation.

As Arthur was putting things away after the class, his fellow instructor, Loretta, came in and asked, 'How did it go?' Arthur replied wearily, 'Some of them are doing fine, but I'm afraid at least half of them will never pass the practical on Friday.' He added with determination, 'I guess I'll just have to go on showing them how again and again until they all catch on.'

As you analyze this case, please assume that while he agreed such things as learning to prevent heart disease were important, Arthur's highest priority during these classes was to help students learn to actually perform the four procedures correctly and with confidence. In terms of that objective:

1. Do you think Arthur made good use of demonstrations and verbal instructions to provide students with a clear, easily-remembered mental image of how the procedures should be performed?
2. Did he use return demonstrations effectively? Did he provide sufficient opportunities for each student to have the amount and type of practice and feedback they needed to master execution of the procedures?
3. Were the telling, showing and doing components of instruction sensibly related to each other? Was their timing logical? Was the demonstration done in a way that made imitation by the student easy?
4. What would you have done differently if you had been the instructor?

FEEDBACK ON EXERCISE 15

This instructor's initial use of demonstrations and verbal instructions had many strong points.

- Use of a motion picture at the very beginning gave the students a good overall image of the procedures to serve as an organizing framework for the more detailed information that followed. This is a procedure in which motion and timing are important, so still pictures or verbal descriptions alone would probably be less effective. The use of animation helped emphasize key points and encouraged students to begin to develop a list of procedural cues. Portrayal of a successful resuscitation in the film was probably reassuring. The filmed demonstrations on human subjects may have been more skilled, interesting and realistic than the demonstrations a novice instructor could provide with a mannikin.

- In his follow-up demonstrations Arthur helped students make the transition to the equipment they would use in practice, and provided further emphasis on key points in procedure and use of verbal cues.

- The printed booklets relieved students of the need for extensive note-taking, and provided an accurate reference for use at home. They also placed strong emphasis on verbal cues and related these cues to visual images of steps in the procedure through use of diagrams and drawings.

- The first class was largely free of irrelevant instruction. The filmed descriptions of anatomy and physiology were directly tied to CPR procedure, and should help many students understand enough about how CPR works to let them use logic to recall steps in performance. Although learning about prevention of heart disease, and appropriate management of the mannikins were not Arthur's primary objectives, these are valuable parts of the overall course and were covered without excessive use of time.

The fine work done by the American Heart Association on development of instructional materials for CPR training certainly paid off here by making the information-giving (showing and telling) segment of the course relevant, organized, interesting and efficient.

The return demonstration segments of the course also had a number of potential strengths:

- Use of simulator mannikins allowed the students to practice and get feedback on performance of several components of the procedure that require development of sensorimotor skills and cannot safely be practiced on a classmate.

- Ample time was planned for 'hand-on' sessions (3 of the first 4 hours of class were scheduled for this.)

- Dividing the class of 25 into two groups for practice made it easier for instructors to give individualized guidance and feedback.

However, Arthur's use of these promising opportunities for practice was disappointing.

- He began by using a large part of the time set aside for student practice to repeat a demonstration that was almost identical to the one the students had just seen in the film. By the time he was finished with this and several other bits of probably unnecessary 'telling', only 14 minutes remained for student practice the first day.

- Because most practice was concentrated on work with the two mannikins, many students spent much of their time during the 'hands on' periods standing around watching one another in an unstructured way, and waiting for a turn.

- Practice, when it did occur, was quite unorganized. Students were given no advice on what to practice first, and seemed to be simply trying different things on a hit or miss basis.

- Although the pressure gauge on the adult mannikin did give students feedback on the force of their chest compressions, and Arthur tried to move from student to student as practice took place, many parts of each student's performance were probably not evaluated or reinforced. This deficiency was caused in part by Arthur's failure to encourage or assist the students to assess their own or each other's performance. Some students probably helped each other spontaneously, but others may have felt entirely dependent on Arthur for feedback.

Arthur also did very little to help the students make the transition from seeing to doing. For example,

- The case summary does not tell what camera angles were used during the filmed demonstrations of the CPR procedures, but we do know that Arthur gave his demonstrations in the center of the room with students observing from all sides. This means that many of them were viewing his performance from an angle that was very dissimilar to the one from which they would observe their own actions. Students who stood at the head of the mannikin, for example, would need to convert left to right and top to bottom in translating their observations of Arthur's chest compressions into a visual image of their own actions. Such reversals can be a significant impediment to learning a complex new motor skill.

- Both the film and Arthur's demonstrations covered four very different procedures—each of them quite complex. This meant, for example, that students who began the practice session by attempting to position themselves for the one-man CPR procedure had to separate out the words and images they had been given for that technique from the similar yet different cues for three other procedures.

- However, there was one even more serious obstacle to effective practice for most students—the long delay that took place between their observation of the filmed and live demonstrations and the time when they were finally able to try performing the procedures themselves. For some students this delayed imitation did not take place until two days later. Arthur's vague recommendation that they 'study their booklets at home' did little to bridge this gap.

Small wonder that when the students finally did have a chance to practice, Arthur observed a serious amount of confusion and error. Unfortunately, his response was to take still more of the practice time to doggedly repeat the demonstrations.

You may have identified a wide variety of ways in which this potentially excellent course could be improved. Here are a few suggestions to compare with your own. Most of them concern changes in the way Arthur handled the practice sessions.

1. During his own demonstrations of the procedures Arthur could:

- ask the students to position themselves so they could observe his performance at least part of the time from the 'point of view of the performer'. This might mean they would need to take turns standing behind him to look over his shoulder. This would be especially worthwhile if Arthur explicitly asked the students to try to imagine it was their own hands and body position they were observing, i.e. to do mental practice of the procedure as they watched.

- ask the students to actively rehearse the verbal cues associated with each step in the procedure as they watched his performance. He might ask them to 'tell me what to do next' or to 'tell me what I'm doing now' or simply to 'think silently to yourself — what am I doing? What words did the film use to describe this step?'

2. He could break his demonstrations into smaller parts by alternating short periods of demonstration and practice and working on only one procedure at a time. This would reduce the confusion of trying to master several procedures at once, and greatly shorten the delay between seeing and doing each procedure.

3. During the return demonstration periods Arthur could increase the amount of practice and feedback each student is allowed by:

   • dividing each of the complex procedures into a series of component subroutines, and having students practice each of these separately until they could do it correctly.

   • allowing them to practice as many of these subroutines as possible by working with a partner rather than the mannikin. Only a few parts of the total procedure really require the mannikin for safe practice (e.g. chest compressions and mouth-to-mouth breathing). Other steps can be practiced as well or even better on a classmate (e.g. checking pulse and breathing, positioning the 'victim'). This should make it unnecessary for any student to spend much time simply waiting and watching.

   • providing a specific list of things to check in the performance of each subroutine and asking students to assess their own work and that of their partner.

4. Arthur could also reduce the students' uncertainty about what they are supposed to do during practice periods, and make sure each student really does practice all of the procedures, by providing a more organized structure for practice and clearer instructions. This could be done in several different ways. For example, Arthur could:

   • set up a series of different practice stations, each with a written list of instructions for practice of a different subroutine or procedure, and each with a set of written guidelines for evaluating performance of that component. Students could then be asked to rotate through each of these stations
   or
   • Arthur could demonstrate one part of a procedure or subroutine that does not require a mannikin for practice and then immediately have all students practice that component with a partner before going on to another subroutine.

5. Arthur will still need to find a way for each student to practice with the mannikin, and some of this practice must come after all the subroutines have been learned and the student is ready to try putting the pieces together. Even if we assume that the Center cannot arrange to buy, rent or borrow additional mannikins, there are several ways in which Arthur might reduce the bottleneck the need for mannikin practice is likely to present near the end of the second class.

   • He could look for students who master the subroutines quickly and move them to the mannikins for practice of the integrated procedure as early as possible. This would free mannikin time for other students at the end of class, and might enable Arthur to enlist the first students as assistant teachers.

   • Near the end of the second class, the size of practice groups at the mannikin stations could be increased to 3 or 4. While one student actually performs the total procedure, the others could be actively involved by asking them to do 'mental practice' or covert rehearsal of the same procedure. Once they have had some physical experience in doing each of the subroutines, most students should be able to imagine themselves going through the full procedure: counting compressions, changing position, checking for pulse and so forth at the pace and rhythm required for correct performance. The same sort of imaginary drill could be carried out by students at home in preparation for their final practical test. The booklet could then serve as a reference for checking their memory of the procedure, instead of something they simply read and re-read in an unstructured way.

- Arthur might also explore the possibility of juggling schedules with the practice group working with the second instructor. If he and his fellow teacher could arrange to use the mannikins at different times, each group might be able to double its available resources of simulators.

These specific suggestions for improvement are only examples. However, they do incorporate some general principles that have very broad application. Stated simply, some **guidelines** worth considering in many demonstrations include:

1. Begin by giving students a clear, visual picture of the overall procedure they are about to learn.

2. When more detailed demonstration begins, don't present too much at one time. Break complex procedures into subroutines students can work on one at a time.

3. Let students observe from a point of view that makes it easy for them to visualize their own performance.

4. Let students imitate what they have seen with a minimum of delay.

5. Emphasize selected, key points in performance and give students short verbal cues to help them remember these steps.

6. Don't clutter up your performance instructions with unnecessary explanations.

7. Do explain enough about why the procedure is done in the recommended way to help students figure out what to do if they forget a step.

8. Provide back-up instructions in writing, using terms the students can understand and use as verbal cues.

9. Provide plenty of feedback, especially in early stages of practice by the student — and add to what you provide by helping students learn to assess their own performance.

10. As learning progresses, place greater emphasis on how the performance should feel if it is correct and less on verbal cues.

OBSERVATION

One of the greatest advantages of clinical teaching is the opportunity it provides for students to observe real people doing real things. In the classroom the instructor can show films, assign readings, schedule role playing and describe her own experiences to help students visualize clinical events. However, these activities may be troublesome to arrange and often provide only a pale image of reality. In the clinic the teacher can easily take advantage of activities that are part of the facility's regular operations to provide students with a wide range of rich and authentic experiences.

For fieldwork students and staff trainees observational experiences are especially important and varied. In the space of a few weeks, for example, a single student might be:

- sent to pathology to observe an autopsy

- taken to watch while their supervisor interviews a difficult client

- asked to sit in on a discharge planning conference

- assigned to spend a day accompanying a staff member on home visits

- and scheduled to accompany a patient as he undergoes a special diagnostic procedure.

Clinical observation is somewhat less important in patient education, since the real world for which the patient is preparing lies outside the hospital or clinic walls. However, sometimes patients and their families also can profit from observing as other patients use the techniques they need to learn and cope with the problems they will confront.

The purposes of observation can be as varied as its content; however the most common uses fall into the following five broad categories:

A. To assist the student *to explore unfamiliar options and identify personal interests.* Patients, staff and students sometimes need to make important choices among options for learning that are so unfamiliar that sensible selection is difficult. Sampling these options through brief observation can help to reduce the mystery and let students decide more realistically what they want to learn and how they prefer to learn it.

B. *To provide a foundation for later, more specific instruction.* Observation can be used early in training to help students get a general picture of something that is unfamiliar, complicated and difficult to describe in words alone. Even though they may not fully understand some of what they see, such early encounters with reality can help students:

- visualize the main components of a complex procedure or situation

- anticipate the kinds of responsibilities and relationships they will have in the future

- recognize the value of areas of study they might otherwise regard as boring or unimportant

- overcome misconceptions, fears, or dislikes based on ignorance or poor past experiences.

C. *To improve specific judgmental, planning or communication skills.* Observations can be used to let students practice a wide variety of intellectual skills. As he watches, the student can attempt to:

- decide what he would do or say if he were an active player in the scene he is observing

- use theories he has learned earlier to classify, analyze or explain the specific events he sees

- identify problems, compare approaches, predict outcomes or react in any of a number of different ways to the things he observes.

D. To help the student *build a mental data base* of the range and pattern of variations that can occur within a single clinical problem. The novice student, staff member or patient usually has only a limited amount of first-hand experience on which to base judgments about whether a problem is serious or whether the way it is responding to treatment is adequate. Observations can be an efficient method for broadening that experience and help to make the student's expectations realistic.

E. To help the student *get fresh ideas* and consider different approaches to dealing with or interpreting a familiar problem. Even highly experienced staff, patients and students can profit from observing the work of others. By allowing them to compare their own methods with what they see others do observations can rekindle enthusiasm and serve as an antidote for 'tunnel vision'.

To achieve such a wide variety of purposes observations must be designed in an equally wide variety of ways. However, the following general factors are important common denominators in planning for most of these experiences.

1. During most observations the student is a spectator, not a participant. Although he may be given a few simple tasks in order to make his presence seem natural, the observer usually is not expected to take responsibility for any of the major events that occur.

2. This does not mean the observer needs to be inactive. It simply means his activities are covert. He is expected to notice without pointing, worry without frowning, judge without speaking, and plan without stepping forward to present or implement his plan.

3. The events the observer watches are not taking place primarily for his benefit, and often cannot be manipulated to make the elements that are most significant for his learning stand out. Many different things may attract the observer's attention and stimulate his thinking. Some of these will be relevant for learning, others may be simply distractions or diversions.

4. To help students make good use of these abundant stimuli, the instructor must try to anticipate what kinds of things the student will witness during the observation, and must decide to which of these she hopes the student will give greatest attention. Then the instructor must plan practical methods for structuring the student's activity during the observation to encourage the focus that will be most useful.

5. Unlike many other instructional activities, the instructor must guide the student's attention during observations primarily through things she does before the observation begins or after it is finished. The instructor frequently is not present during the experience; and, even if she is with the student, circumstances usually make it inappropriate for her to question, explain or point out to the students the events of greatest significance.

Planning for observation thus begins, as does all good instructional planning, with an attempt to select important instructional objectives in one or more of the general categories described earlier. Once the instructor has thought of a situation in which the student's mastery of these objectives might be stimulated by observing real events, she can begin to decide how to help the student get the most out of this opportunity.

To see how this works in practice, try your hand at planning for the student in the following exercise.

HELPING STUDENTS LEARN ON THEIR OWN: THE CASE OF THE WIDE-EYED OBSERVER

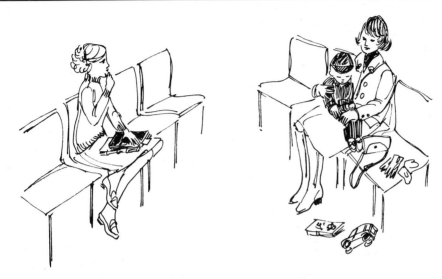

Marjorie Frederick is in the final year of a social work program at a large university, and doing clinical fieldwork at the university's medical center. This morning her supervisor arranged for Marjorie to spend an hour and a half observing in the pediatric oncology out-patient clinic. It is attended principally by children with leukemia who come in frequently for chemotherapy and evaluation. Because the children sometimes have to wait to see the doctor, the staff have converted one end of the clinic waiting room into a play area. It is equipped with a number of well-worn books and a few simple toys such as trucks and blocks. The area is used both by many of the patients and by healthy pre-school brothers and sisters who sometimes also come with the parent. Many of the mothers and fathers have gotten to know each other through their frequent visits, and one of the nurses or a social worker assigned to this clinic is often in the area talking with a parent or playing with a child. It is a busy and rather crowded place.

Marjorie's supervisor scheduled this observation as part of her pediatric experience and discussed it in advance with the clinic staff to make sure they were willing to have a student observer. On the morning of the observation the supervisor accompanied Marjorie to the clinic, introduced her to the nurse in charge, and suggested she spend most of her time in the waiting room observing the patients, their families and the staff. After taking a quick tour of the examining rooms with the senior nurse, and meeting the physician and his resident, Marjorie spent the rest of the time sitting in the waiting room. Towards the end of the morning she chatted with several of the mothers and with a patient who asked if she could fix a loose wheel on his truck.

By the time her assigned observation was over it was time for lunch. Marjorie met one of her classmates in the cafeteria and her friend asked, 'What happened to you this morning? I didn't see you in the office.' 'Well, I was up in the pediatric oncology clinic observing most of the morning', Marjorie replied. 'I've never been there. Was it interesting?' her friend asked. 'I guess so', Marjorie said uncertainly. 'At first I felt kind of funny because I didn't really have anything to do, and I wasn't sure what I was supposed to get out of it. Then one of the mothers asked if my child was in for treatment, and I had to explain I was just a student.' Marjorie paused, and then went on, 'I guess the whole scene really got me. The mothers are so worried and trying so hard to be brave, and the kids look so sick. There are so many of them: a couple of them didn't even have enough energy to play, they just sat on their mother's laps, and lots of them wear little baseball caps to hide their bald heads . . . I'll sure never forget it!'

Instructions for working with this case:

We really can't tell what Marjorie learned from this observation—or what her supervisor intended her to learn. This brief description tells us nothing about the instructional objectives and only a little about what Marjorie noticed, thought and felt during her observation. However, the case does provide information you can use to do some instructional planning of your own.

Imagine that you are Marjorie's supervisor. If you are not a social worker and would prefer to plan for a student in your own field, go ahead and make that change, but please keep the instructional situation the same.

Write down your ideas as you work on the following two tasks. If possible, try to exchange your work with at least one other clinical teacher who also does this exercise. If you work alone write your ideas down anyway. This will make it easier for you to evaluate them objectively when you read the feedback section.

TASK A Establish a purpose for this observation

What do you think Marjorie could learn from observing in this particular waiting room for an hour and a half? Be as specific as you can in writing down at least one instructional objective you think this experience could help Marjorie achieve.

TASK B Decide how you would structure this experience

As the student's instructor, what would you plan to do to help her achieve this particular objective? Please assume that you will *not* be with the student during the observation period itself. Write down a list of any specific things you would do before and/or after her observation to help make sure the experience is worthwhile.

FEEDBACK

FEEDBACK ON EXERCISE 16

Even fairly commonplace clinical situations, such as this waiting room, provide such a variety of different stimuli that they can serve as a location for work on many different instructional objectives. There is no single set of best objectives and no one best method of structuring such an observation. The important thing is that there be some clearly defined purpose for the student's activity, and that it be structured in a way that is logically related to that purpose. The following four steps should help you review the soundness of your own plans.

1. Begin by thinking about whether the objective you selected for this exercise is defined clearly enough to provide the focus needed for planning. One way to do this is to see if you can classify your objective using the five broad categories of purpose listed on page 143 of this section. If you are working with a group of colleagues or a partner, decide which of the five categories best describes your objective. Then exchange objectives with someone else who is doing this exercise and see whether you agree on the classification. Putting your objective into a category is not a necessary part of planning, but for the purpose of this exercise it will make it easier for you to judge what sort of structure is called for, and it can help you decide whether your objective is specific enough to serve as the basis for further planning. If you have difficulty classifying your objective, this may be simply because you have been imaginative and selected a worthwhile purpose for this observation that was not thought of by the author of this Handbook. However, you should also ask yourself whether the problem stems from having too vague an idea of purpose. For example, if you answered the first question for this case by simply saying you wanted the student to 'be exposed to oncology' or to 'find out about pediatrics', your purpose is probably still too general to help you much in designing a worthwhile observation.

2. Next, try to analyze the overall approach you took to providing structure by comparing what you planned to do before or after the observation with the following two general methods of instruction.

The first, and probably most familiar, is a method in which most of the structure is determined by the teacher, and students are given a set of specific instructions or a conceptual framework to guide their thinking at the very beginning of the experience. This approach to teaching has application to many other types of instruction besides observations, and has been given various labels in the education literature. Here we will call it the *expository model* of teaching to emphasize the teacher's role in explaining, defining and providing an interpretative framework for the student to use in thinking about the events he observes. You could provide such structure before the observation began, using either or both of two special techniques:

Pre-sets: instructions that *direct the student's attention* to specific aspects of the situation he observes. For example, you might plan to say to Marjorie:

— 'Pay special attention to the way the nurses interact with the mothers.'

— 'See if you think there are any differences in the play activities the patients choose and what the normal brothers and sisters seem to prefer.'

— 'Think about how you would feel about the physical and social arrangements in this waiting room if you were one of the mothers.'

Advance organizers. These do more than just tell the student what to notice, they also *provide an organizational framework or system* the student can use to process or store the specific information, ideas or feelings that are generated by the real events he encounters during the observation. These organizers may be general theories, systems of classification, procedural guidelines or concepts and principles that provide what Ausubel has called 'intellectual scaffolding' for subsequent experiences.[1] By the time they reach the clinic, students often have already acquired theoretical knowledge that can serve this purpose. However, the clinical instructor may want to remind the students to use specific theories or review relevant theory with them before the observation starts. For example, the day before she went to the clinic to observe, you could say to Marjorie, 'I'd like you to use Talcott Parsons' theory of the sick role to analyze the interactions you see between the children and their mothers. Think about how accurately that theory seems to predict the specific things you see the mothers and children do and say. Look for actions that do seem to fit the theory and for any that do not. It won't be appropriate for you to take notes while you're there, but try to remember some specific examples so we can talk about them later. I know you studied Parsons at school last year, but if you're not sure you remember all the details of his theory you might want to review your class notes before you go to clinic.' Notice that in this sample of preparatory instructions the student is given a series of specific questions to attempt to answer during the observation, questions that call for a specific type of thinking as well as for use of a specific theoretical framework. Alternatively, you might ask the student to use theory for some quite different purpose, such as to develop a plan of action or formulate hypotheses about what was causing the events she observed. Whatever emphasis you choose, the advance organizer will have the most powerful directive effect on the student's thinking if you not only suggest concepts that are relevant to the observed situation but also tell the student how these concepts are to be used. Simply telling Marjorie to 'think about the way Talcott Parsons defined the sick role while you're in clinic this morning' will provide some direction for her thinking, but does not help her understand exactly what this 'thinking' should involve.

Of course, this may be exactly what you want—for the student to decide for herself what is significant in this situation, and how her observations can be organized and interpreted. In that case, you would be likely to choose the second general approach. It too can be used in many types of teaching, and has been given a variety of names: experiential learning, inquiry training, learning by discovery, training in inductive thinking. Here we will call it the *discovery model* to emphasize the student's freedom to invent for himself the conceptual framework and processes he uses to react to the specific events he sees during observation. In this model, experience precedes theory and provides the substance out of which the student develops his own concepts, definitions and explanations. Real events are analyzed retrospectively to generate ideas that help to describe and explain the experience in some systematic way. In its most student-directed form, this approach restricts the instructor from even hinting at a pre-set or advance organizer; and it also prohibits the instructor from asking deliberately 'leading questions' to help the student arrive at the 'right' interpretation when the observation is over. This does not mean the instructor must be entirely uncritical of the student's theoretical structuring of his experiences. For example, if the student is attempting to propose hypotheses that explain what he saw, and these seem to be inconsistent with some of the events he reports, the instructor can point out these inconsistencies. If the concepts or labels the student proposes are so incompletely defined no one else can understand them, the instructor may probe for clarification. However, in this approach the emphasis is on the quality of the student's inquiry process, not on whether the student makes good use of a specific set of ideas proposed by the instructor.

Each of these models has many variations, and in some cases they can be combined to create an intermediate method in which the instructor and student share responsibility for determining focus and process. For example, you might plan to use only a very general pre-set before the observation and then to follow the observation with a discussion based on carefully planned leading questions designed to encourage Marjorie to search her knowledge of general theory for principles that could explain what she observed.

3. Each of the two general models is useful, but they are useful for achieving somewhat different purposes. Once you have decided which elements of the models you plan to use, go back to your objective and think about whether the method of structuring you chose is logically matched to that goal.

Some goals can be achieved using either of the two models. For example, if your objective was for Marjorie to learn to anticipate more accurately the types of responsibilities she might have if she were to work in a pediatric clinic, you might tell her in advance this was what you hoped she would think about during the observation; or you could wait until the experience was over to see what Marjorie noticed about staff duties on her own and then ask questions to help clarify and generalize these observations. If you wanted her to learn to use theory to explain changes in the children's physical appearance, you could tell her what theories to use and send her to the observation equipped with a set of questions to guide her thinking; or you could wait until after the observation was over and use a different sort of question to encourage her to discover her own logical explanations of the changes she noticed without being prompted.

Other goals, however, can probably be achieved more fully or more efficiently using one approach rather than the other. For example, if your primary purpose were for Marjorie to expand her knowledge of the frequency with which certain side-effects occur after chemotherapy, it would probably be a mistake to say nothing and hope that this would be something she would notice during the observation. She might do so, but without any advance direction it seems likely she might put all her effort into thinking about some of the many other aspects of this complex situation, and come away with very little impression of what side-effects could be observed. By contrast, if your intent is for Marjorie to improve her ability to identify problems or set treatment priorities for herself, you will only defeat your purpose if you structure her observation by telling her at the outset what problems and priorities you believe deserve greatest attention.

As you review your own plans for purpose and structure, try to be realistic in deciding whether what you propose will really work. Will the student notice the things you are sending her to see if you give her no advance direction? If you want the student to unscramble ambiguous situations for herself, have you allowed her the freedom to do this?

4. Finally, think for a moment about some of the practical matters your plan involves. In the case description Marjorie's supervisor did several things that seemed likely to make the experience go smoothly. For example, she scheduled the observation in advance rather than on the spur of the moment, made sure the clinic staff were willing to have the student observe and that they knew what her role would be, and took time to take Marjorie to the clinic to introduce her. All this should help put the student at ease and make sure she doesn't waste time during the observation worrying about the fact that no one seemed to be expecting her. Depending upon the objective and approach to structuring you selected you might need to do some additional practical things: schedule a follow-up conference, assign Marjorie to review material in a text, provide her with a form to use in tabulating observations. Even if no such practical arrangements are needed, you should plan to do one thing Marjorie's supervisor neglected — give her at least a general idea of what she is supposed to get out of this experience. If you plan to use the expository method this will be an explicit part of your plan, but use of the discovery model need not be accompanied by secrecy or mystery. If you want the student to decide for herself what is interesting, to select her own approach to thinking about what she observes, tell her this is what you have in mind. Telling a student she is free to chart her own course is not limiting or directive, and it can keep the student from wasting valuable time during the observation trying to guess why on earth you arranged for her to be there.

SUPERVISED PRACTICE

Practice under supervision provides an important bridge between didactic instruction and independent use of a clinical skill. During these sessions the instructor serves as observer, coach and troubleshooter. Although he may interrupt the student's work from time to time to repeat instructions, make suggestions or explain something that has happened, the instructor's main responsibility is not to present information—it is to help the student learn by doing. This help can take a variety of forms: reassurance, cues, reinforcement: and protective help if things go wrong. Chapter 1 of this Handbook includes a discussion of strategies for providing reinforcement. In this section our concern will be chiefly with planning for the scope and difficulty of the tasks to be performed during practice, and with methods for providing cues while practice is under way.

We should begin by conceding that supervised practice is often an intimidating experience for students. This may be true even when the student is unsure of his own skills and wants the instructor's advice and support. Few of us are truly at ease when someone is looking over our shoulder—however benevolently. If the student's work involves interaction with a third person the instructor's presence may also intrude on and disrupt that relationship. To be an effective coach, therefore, the instructor must find ways to help without interfering or threatening. He must try to meet the following challenges:

1. To be close enough to the action to observe accurately and give help quickly if help is needed, without making his presence so noticeable or unnatural that it distracts the student and makes people with whom the student is working uneasy.

2. To provide sufficient guidance to help the student avoid mistakes that are risky, frustrating, confusing, or waste a great deal of time, without intervening unnecessarily and depriving the student of a chance to work through problems himself.

3. To keep the scope and difficulty of assigned tasks within the student's present capabilities, without fragmenting or simplifying them so much the student's experience is unrealistic.

As with other methods of instruction, supervised practice is most likely to be satisfying and instructive if it is based on sensible planning. The following exercise illustrates some of the factors planning for supervised practice often needs to take into account.

SUPERVISING PRACTICE OF A COMPLEX SKILL: THE CASE OF THE FLUSTERED TECHNICIAN

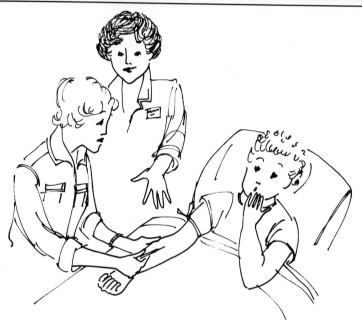

Patricia White is a 19-year-old student in an on-the-job training program for laboratory technicians at Central City Hospital. She began training a month after completing secondary school, and has done well in the program so far. Pat enjoys the work and feels it will be much more rewarding than any of her earlier part-time jobs babysitting, selling tickets at a movie theatre, and working in a small convenience store. She is a conscientious worker who says very little in class, but is always well prepared if the instructor asks her a question. During the initial part of their training Pat and the other three trainees who started work when she did attended a series of classes and lab sessions in which they learned theory and technique for the basic procedures they will be expected to carry out as part of their jobs. One of these was the procedure for drawing a 5cc blood sample from an adult patient using the median cubital vein (basic phlebotomy technique). At the start of their training the students received a Techniques Notebook which included a detailed step-by-step description of each procedure for which they will be responsible in their jobs. The procedure for phlebotomy technique is attached. In recent classes their instructor has discussed and demonstrated this procedure, and the students have had several opportunities to practice it on one another during labs. In these practice sessions the trainees go through all steps except actually inserting the needle. They take turns playing the part of a patient.

Procedure for phlebotomy technique

Procedure for drawing a 5 cc blood sample from an adult patient using the median cubital vein.*

*Based on a task analysis by Loretta Donald MSN

Steps in performance

1. Introduce yourself to the patient and check his/her identity by asking him/her to state his/her name. On in-patients also check identification bracelet.

2. Explain the purpose of your visit.

3. Talk briefly with patient to determine past experience with this procedure and assess level of anxiety.

4. Ask patient which arm he/she prefers you use, and obtain permission to examine venipuncture site.

5. Have patient sit or lie down with arm supported and expose site.

6. Continue talking with the patient while using finger palpation to check for a suitable site in the ante-cubital area.

7. Decide whether site is suitable.

8. If suitable, monitor patient's expression and continue conversation while quickly attaching needle to vacutainer holder and placing 5 ml vacutainer tube in holder. Do not engage tube and needle. Do this without waving the needle needlessly in front of the patient.

8A. If site *not* suitable, ask to check the other arm and repeat steps 6 and 7. Then do step 8.

9. Place assembled vacutainer, alcohol, dry gauze and tourniquet on the side of the patient from which blood will be drawn. It should be within easy reach but out of the patient's direct view—to one side.

10. Minimize patient's anxiety by assembling materials quickly, maintaining occasional eye contact and continuing conversation.

11. Tie tourniquet on upper 1/3 of arm so you can easily untie it with one hand.

12. Instruct patient to open and close fist several times as you palpate vein for increased pressure, estimating its depth and diameter.

13. Cleanse site with 70% isopropyl alcohol and dry with gauze. Site should be recleansed if contaminated by repalpation.

14. Explain to patient what he/she may feel and allow him/her to watch procedure or look away. (A person's reaction to a procedure often is related to how they control their anxiety.)

15. Pick up the vacutainer assembly with your dominant hand, holding the barrel between your thumb and last three fingers, with your index finger resting against the hub of the needle.

16. With your free hand, support the patient's arm at the elbow, leaving your thumb free to compress and stretch the soft tissues below the puncture site to anchor the vein and pull it taut during needle insertion.

17. Anchoring the back of your fingers on your dominant hand against the patient's arm, insert the needle (bevel up) to enter the vein with a single, direct puncture of skin and vein. Be careful not to exit on opposite side of the vein.

18. Change the vacutainer assembly to the other hand and hold it firmly in place.

19. Gently push the vacutainer tube forward using the flange of the vacutainer holder until the tube is engaged with the base of the needle.

20. Hold assembly in place until tube is filled with blood. Then smoothly disengage tube from the needle and remove it from the holder.

20A. If blood does not enter the tube, slightly pulling back the needle may help. If still unsuccessful, palpate needle and vein, then carefully adjust needle until blood flows.

21. Address patient's reactions by asking, 'How are you feeling?' and stating, 'It's almost finished.'

22. Release tourniquet.

23. Withdraw needle and cover site immediately with a piece of sterile gauze. Apply pressure over insertion site.

24. Place vacutainer assembly and blood sample out of the patient's direct view while assuring the patient that the procedure is finished.

25. Continue to compress site until bleeding stops, then apply a small bandage over the area and ask the patient to leave it in place for the rest of the day.

26. Label the blood sample.

Earlier this week Pat's supervisor, Maria Mercado, checked her performance of the phlebotomy procedure on another trainee. Pat sometimes had to stop and think a moment to recall some of the fine points of a few steps, and was still a little squeamish about the prospect of inserting the needle, but her technical performance seemed acceptable and Maria felt she was ready to begin work with patients. Maria planned to stay with Pat during her first few attempts to take blood samples from patients in order to coach her if needed and to be on hand to help if anything went wrong. Maria felt such direct supervision was needed because this would be Pat's first direct contact with patients since starting training.

This morning Maria took Pat with her to the in-patient surgical units to see several patients for whom blood tests had been ordered. The first patient they saw was a 35-year-old woman who was recovering from a hysterectomy. Maria decided to draw this sample herself to give Pat a chance to review the technique before she tried it. As they entered the room, the patient obviously recognized Maria, smiled, and said, 'Hi, back again? Sorry—you got my last drop of blood the last time.' She laughed and so did Maria as she replied, 'Oh, come on, I'll bet you've still got a little hiding in there somewhere. Which arm would you like me to use?' 'How about this one?' said the patient, holding out her left arm. 'Fine', replied Maria and proceeded to palpate for the vein, prepare the vacutainer, and go through the procedure as outlined in the protocol, chatting with the patient as she did this about a television program they had both watched the night before.

When they were back in the corridor Maria said to Pat, 'Okay. The next one's all yours.' The next patient on their list was Mrs Murdock, a moderately obese, 47-year-old housewife who had been admitted for an elective cholecystectomy. She was sitting in an armchair next to her bed as they entered, reading a magazine. Maria stayed near the door behind the trainee as Pat approached the patient, smiled, and said, 'Good morning. I'm Miss White from the lab.' After checking the patient's identity, Pat explained, 'Your Doctor has asked me to take a blood sample from you.' Mrs Murdock looked at her apprehensively, and asked, 'Does that mean you're going to stick me?' 'Yes,' said Pat, 'I will need to use a needle. Have you had a blood sample taken before?' 'Yes, and it was terrible. I hate needles. The last girl who did this just about killed me, and she left an awful big bruise on my arm. I hope you're not going to do that.' 'It'll be okay,' replied Pat, 'this will just take a minute. Can I get you up on your bed?' I'd like to do this with you lying down.' Mrs Murdock got onto the bed as requested, and Pat began to pull up the sleeve of her bathrobe on the arm nearest her, Mrs Murdock's right arm. At this point, Maria stepped forward and said, 'I think it would be easier if we took her bathrobe off first.' Pat said, 'Oh yes. Would you sit up please Mrs Murdock?' She helped Mrs Murdock take her right arm out of the sleeve and lie down again, then began to inspect and palpate the antecubital area. Maria stepped forward again and said, 'While we're at it, let's just pull off these slippers so you don't get the bed dirty', and removed Mrs Murdock's slippers. Pat began her inspection once more, bending over Mrs Murdock's arm, looking at it closely, and palpating at several different spots in the area. 'I have terrible veins', Mrs Murdock told her. 'Do you think you can find it?' 'It's okay', said Pat. She then began assembling her equipment on the bedside table. 'That would be a littler easier if you moved it closer' said Maria, and pulled the table nearer to the bed. Mrs Murdock looked at Pat and said, 'Are you a student or something?' Pat hesitated, looked at Maria, and said, 'Well, I work here . . .' Maria stepped forward again and said, 'It's okay. Miss White knows how' and stepped back. Pat then began to apply the tourniquet to Mrs Murdock's arm. She did this carefully and rather slowly, pulling at it several times to change its position slightly. As she completed this and began to palpate the arm again, Maria stepped forward and said, 'Let's just move this a little higher' and unfastened the tourniquet to replace it slightly higher on the arm. Pat then asked Mrs Murdock to make a fist while she began palpating the arm again. After a moment she swabbed the area vigorously with alcohol, dried it with a piece of gauze, slipped her left hand under Mrs Murdock's elbow and reached for the vacutainer apparatus. Just then Mrs Murdock moved and Pat hit the table, knocking the equipment onto the floor. 'Oh my!' said Pat and Mrs Murdock in unison. Pat began picking up the pieces of the broken vacutainer, but Maria intervened saying, 'Just leave that for now. Here's a new one. We can take care of the other one later.' 'Please. Couldn't you do this?' asked Mrs Murdock, looking at Maria. 'No, it's okay. Go ahead Pat. Now please, Mrs Murdock, try not to move.' said Maria, giving Pat a reassuring look. Pat began again using the new vacutainer, and succeeded in inserting the needle, but no blood appeared as she began to withdraw the plunger. 'Try withdrawing it a little', Maria suggested, 'and Mrs Murdock, see if you can relax a little. This won't take long now.' Pat realigned the needle but was still unsuccessful in getting blood. 'Oh, I can't stand this!' said Mrs. Murdock, 'You'll just have to do it.' 'Okay', replied Maria. Pat stepped aside in relief, and Maria took over.

As you review this case, try to identify:

1. any specific things the supervisor did that you feel were probably helpful to the trainee in her attempt to carry out this procedure with a patient for the first time and in her learning of the procedure.

2. any things you would have
   * done differently,
   * omitted, or
   * added
   if you had been the supervisor.

If you are not familiar with the phlebotomy technique, don't worry. Assume the step-by-step description in the protocol is correct and concentrate on the supervisor's teaching technique rather than on the fine points of drawing a blood sample.

FEEDBACK ON EXERCISE 17

To review your reactions to this case, think about them in relation to the points emphasized in the introductory pages of this section.

1. How to be available without being disruptive

Maria's decision to provide direct supervision throughout this student activity seems sensible. Students don't always need continuous, direct supervision the first time they carry out a new procedure, but in this case the procedure is one that could be unpleasant or risky for the patient if key steps are done incorrectly, and assessment of the student's lab performance makes it seem possible she will need help.

However, the supervisor did several things that probably made her presence more disruptive than necessary for both student and patient. For example:

- The supervisor made no effort to introduce herself or explain her presence to the patient when she and Pat entered the room. Hospitalized patients do learn to put up with a series of unannounced people coming in and out of their rooms, but this did little to reassure an already anxious patient. Identification badges and name tags can help patients find out who's who, but a simple, gracious introduction by the supervisor could have helped this encounter get off to a smooth start. As an alternative, the supervisor might have tried to arrange for this student experience to take place in an out-patient area in which she could be on hand in the same room to observe and help if needed, while working with another patient or carrying out some other appropriate task. In that case, the supervisor would only need to explain her presence if she found it necessary to intervene.

- Both the timing and wording of the supervisor's suggestions called attention to the student's inexperience. Although Maria did this in a positive and pleasant manner, her help could have been made less obvious in a variety of ways. For example:

  — Some suggestions could have been worded as questions or phrased in some way that showed Pat was 'in charge' of this procedure. (For example, 'Would you like me to help you get that robe off?')

  — Some could have been made non-verbally. This would be easier if the supervisor stood somewhere other than behind the student, where she is directly in the patient's line of vision. For example, if Maria had stood on the other side of the bed, she probably could have given Pat some unspoken cues and supportive looks without this being obvious to Mrs Murdock.

  — Several of the minor problems Maria mentioned could have been ignored entirely or left for discussion privately with the student after the procedure was completed. Such actions as removing the patient's shoes and repositioning the table really didn't seem necessary, and they challenged the student's competence early in the procedure. It may seem unlikely that any supervisor would make so many unnecessary interruptions, but in actual practice even an experienced teacher may lose sight of her own actions and fail to realize that what was intended as help has become harrassment.

2. How quickly to intervene when a problem does require correction

By the time she had dropped the first vacutainer, the student was probably so thoroughly flustered that she needed immediate, firm direction from her supervisor. In the early stages of the procedure, however, the student might have been less threatened and had a greater opportunity to learn if she had been allowed time to work through some of the simple problems for herself. One of the skills that characterizes a good supervisor is the ability to bite her tongue and wait to see if students will notice and correct problems on their own. You may also have felt the supervisor should have reached some sort of simple agreement with the student in advance about when and how she would provide help. For example, saying to the student, 'I'll be there if you need me, but I won't do anything unless you ask for advice or I see something I think is a real problem' would be more honest than telling the student, 'The next patient is all yours', and then interrupting with a series of unsolicited suggestions.

3. At what level of difficulty should the student be assigned clinical tasks

The supervisor in this case did several good things to ensure that the student was competent to carry out this particular task with a patient. Use of a step-by-step task analysis as the basis for teaching, and assessment in the practice lab provided Pat with a clear picture of what she would be expected to do. It also helped to emphasize the need for good communication with the patient, an aspect of care that can be very fuzzy for an inexperienced student unless it is clearly described. By allowing the student to observe as she carried out the procedure on the first patient, Maria gave the student a timely opportunity to review the component steps and provided a model of interaction that complemented the somewhat artificial portrayal the student had experienced during the role playing in the practice lab.

However, although Pat's performance in the practice lab seemed acceptable, the problems she encountered in working with Mrs Murdock suggest something about this assignment made it too difficult for her. The most likely explanation is that she was unprepared to cope with an anxious patient at the same time as she used her still very new technical skills. You might feel that if her supervisor were more patient and supportive during the early stages of Pat's work with Mrs Murdock this would make it possible for her to complete the procedure without serious problems. For a trainee who is generally poised and at ease with strangers that does seem likely. However, since Pat's behavior in class is somewhat submissive and her earlier work experience has provided little experience in working with anxious adults, additional simplification may be called for. One approach might be to require additional laboratory practice and a higher demonstrated level of technical skill before permitting Pat to attempt the procedure with patients. However, if the other trainees are ready to move on to other techniques, this may prove impractical. In any case, for such additional practice with classmates to be really helpful it would need to include considerable emphasis on communication and patient support techniques.

You might also have identified a number of other ways in which this early clinical experience might have been simplified to make it more appropriate for the student at this point in her training.

For example this might be done:

- by selecting the patient more carefully. For instance, if Maria had simply switched the order of the two patients, she would have had a better opportunity to demonstrate how to reassure an anxious patient, and the student could have made her first attempt to draw a blood sample from an experienced and calm patient.

- by arranging for the student to have her first direct contact with a patient in the course of carrying out some less technically demanding procedure.

- by sharing responsibility with the student for carrying out the total procedure. Since this was the student's first attempt, the supervisor might explain the procedure to the patient and do the needle insertion herself, while asking the student simply to arrange the equipment, select the site, prepare the skin, and apply the tourniquet.

Whatever methods you prefer for modifying supervision or simplifying the procedure, some effort is needed to increase the student's chances of success in this early clinical experience. Both patient and student obviously will survive this encounter, but such unhappy experiences should be avoided if at all possible. Particularly at an early stage in clinical work, this sort of 'public failure' can make students so anxious about working with patients and being supervised that some of their subsequent experiences are largely wasted. Caution at this stage can be a good investment.

Of course, even with careful planning and sensitive guidance, sometimes serious problems arise during supervised practice. When this happens, the supervisor is faced with the difficult decision of whether to insist the student try again, or to take over and finish the job herself. You may have felt Maria was correct in putting the patient's comfort first and completing the procedure for Pat. Or, you may have felt this was unnecessary and that the student deserved another chance to try to complete it successfully herself. A wise decision depends a great deal upon your ability to make an accurate on-the-spot assessment of both the patient's and the student's ability to cope with additional stress. Whichever course of action the supervisor chooses, she will need to follow the procedure with some sort of positive acknowledgment of the patient's help, and with at least a brief, private conference with the student. The student's future progress towards the confidence and competence needed for independent practice will go more smoothly if this experience is ended with reassurance that her errors were not unusual, and with practical planning for future work on specific problem areas.

The example given in this case was that of a staff trainee; however the challenges of providing good direct supervision are much the same for work with patients and their families. Particularly when an important task is being attempted for the first time, the clinical teacher needs to plan carefully to ensure the early success that leads to growing confidence and early independence.

QUESTIONS AND CONFERENCES

In the course of their training, students, staff and patients have many important learning experiences that are not directly supervised by a clinical teacher. Some of these independent activities are planned and scheduled by the teacher, others occur spontaneously; but all can be made more fruitful for the student if they are combined with a well-planned supervisory conference.

Individual conferences with students serve multiple purposes. They may be used to:

- *plan future instructional experiences* by involving students in selection of goals and design of activities

- *share useful information* the student will need in order to carry out independent activities

- *provide an organizing framework* that directs the student's attention and guides his thinking when the activity takes place

- *give students feedback* on the appropriateness and effectiveness of actions they report.

- *extend the learning that occurred during an independent activity* by reflecting on and analyzing what took place in a systematic way.

Effective use of individual conferences obviously calls for a wide range of different teaching skills. Other sections of this Handbook provide suggestions for many of these:

— Chapter 3 presents guidelines for involving students in planning for their own activities through use of *contracting*
— In this chapter, the section on lecturing suggests methods for *selecting* the *information* students need, and the section on observations describes the use of *pre-sets* and *advance organizers* to direct students' attention and structure their thinking, methods frequently used during preparatory conferences.
— Chapter 5 on evaluation includes a section on techniques for giving students *feedback*, an important component of many follow-up conferences.

The bibliographies for those chapters and for this section also provide suggestions for some of the many excellent references you might use to help you go beyond the introductory material presented in this Handbook.

This section, therefore, will be concerned principally with one particular use of individual conferences—to help students extend what they have learned from independent activities.

Kadushin provides a clear description of the purpose and process of individual conferences in his description of supervisory meetings in social work.

The starting point . . . is the report of the worker's activity on the job shared with the supervisor in advance or verbally during the conference. Supervision is 'post facto' teaching . . . The supervisor engages the worker in a systematic, explicit, critical analysis of the work he did and the work he is planning to do . . . The conference is an opportunity for guided self-observation, for systematic introspective–retrospective review of work that has been done, for thinking about the work as 'recollected in tranquillity'.[2]

The instructor's part in helping the student review and learn from this reflection is complex. These conferences are far more than simply a time when students are expected to report what they have done and seen so the instructor can evaluate their work and tell them how to interpret their observations. As Kadushin comments, often 'Experience is fragmented and seemingly chaotic. The supervisor helps the supervisee impose some order and meaning on experience . . . The supervisor does this by asking questions, requesting clarification, freeing, supporting, stimulating, affirming, directing, challenging, and supplementing the worker's thinking.'[2]

At the heart of this process are the instructor's guiding questions. They help to determine which features of the experience will receive most attention, and how the student will attempt to think about or react to those events. Through her questions the instructor can lead the student to search his memory of the experience for trends and patterns in events, gaps and inconsistencies in actions, evidence that supports or challenges his expectations. The instructor can ask the student to recall reactions, describe interpretations, compare interventions, evaluate results, identify problems, formulate hypotheses, clarify explanations, propose action, and analyze the assumptions and motives underlying his own actions. Since the purpose of the conference is to help the student learn, the instructor's decisions about what types of questions to ask should be based on an analysis of which of these many different types of thinking the student most needs to practice.

Some of the questions may be asked early in the conference to give it initial focus and direction. Others may come later as follow-up probes or in response to a student question or comment. In either case, the focus of the questions and the way they are worded will have a powerful influence on what the student learns from the experience and how much.

The need for both the art and science of teaching is very conspicuous in these individual conferences. The medium through which teaching takes place is personal interaction, the often intense give and take, challenge and affirmation, verbal and non-verbal conversation of student and teacher. To do his part in this well, the instructor needs those skills we often think of as the essence of the art of teaching: patience, humor, enthusiasm, sensitivity, honesty, respect for others. Such interaction skills are certainly not without a theoretical base, but they are primarily performing skills, learned through long practice and used in shaping a response to the actions of others in a process that is more often intuitive than deliberate. The instructor can think ahead about the general style that will probably be most helpful, but many of his most important choices about personal interaction can be made only on the spot.

By contrast, a great deal of useful planning can be done in formulating the guiding questions that will provide the intellectual framework for this personal interaction. The instructor can think in advance about:

- why the conference is needed—what she particularly hopes the student will learn from this reflection on experience

- what specific thinking skills or attitudes the student needs in order to achieve these

goals—what she wants to encourage the student to feel or think during the discussion

- how questions can be worded to focus the student's attention on the remembered events of greatest significance and to provoke the thoughts and feelings he needs to practice.

To try to do all this 'off the cuff' while the conference is in progress is unnecessarily risky. Obviously, the instructor will need some ability to think on her feet in order to ask clear and useful questions that follow up on student questions and comments.

The entire discussion cannot be 'scripted' in advance. But even the impromptu questions that may make up large pieces of the conference are more likely to be instructive if they take place within the framework of a well thought-out general plan, and if the instructor has a clear notion of how the wording of questions influences the responses they elicit.

Lest all this sounds as if these conferences must be entirely directed by the instructor and based on a rigid plan that ignores the student's interests and reactions, we should point out that non-directive questioning calls for particularly careful attention to the way instructor questions and comments are worded. This approach to teaching is also based on a clear vision of purpose. To say we want to encourage students to decide for themselves what is important, and to figure out their own solutions to problems, is as definite a statement of purpose as to say we want the student to increase his skill in a particular application of a theory we have decided is useful. Conferences based on such 'liberating' goals require careful wording of questions and comments to encourage the student to think for himself without inadvertently putting the instructor's ideas and preferences in his path.

The following exercise will give you a brief opportunity to practice the sort of question planning good individual conferences require.

EXERCISE 18

USING QUESTIONS TO GUIDE DISCUSSIONS AND CONFERENCES: THE CASE OF THE WANDERING CONVERSATION

Cleo Bryant is a nurse practitioner at a large, urban health maintenance organization. This afternoon she is scheduled to see Olive Dix, a 45-year-old telephone operator who has suffered from severe varicose veins in both legs since her second pregnancy nine years ago. Mrs Dix is nearly 40 pounds overweight and says she has 'been a fatty all my life'. Two months ago she came to the HMO clinic concerned about an unhealed ulcer on the lower part of her left leg. She explained it had developed after she hit her shin on the coffee table, and said it seemed to be getting larger and that she hated the way it looked. After examination and testing Mrs Dix was told the ulcer was the result of poor circulation in her legs. She has received topical treatment for the ulcer and been put on a preventive program to reduce the likelihood of further tissue damage from her circulatory problems. The program includes:

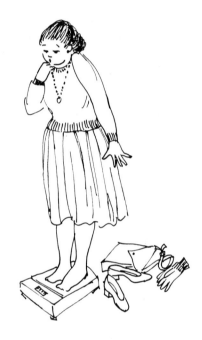

- *instruction in a weight-reduction diet* provided by the HMO's clinical dietitian. Mrs Dix lost 4 pounds during her first month on the diet and was very pleased by this success. She was taught about the food groups and given general guidelines for selecting a balanced, weight-loss diet; but on her last visit reported she 'mostly just eats what's on the sample menus the dietitian gave me. That way I can't make any mistakes'.

- *a recommendation to wear full-length support hose* whenever she is out of bed. She was given a properly fitted set of stockings, taught how to put them on, and urged to do this each day before she gets up. However, Mrs Dix finds the heavyweight surgical hose very uncomfortable, especially on hot days, and says she dislikes the way they look. 'They make me look like more of an elephant than ever!' On her last visit she was given a second pair of lighter weight stockings with the understanding that she will wear these only on special occasions and at times when she does not need to be on her feet much.

- *an explanation of why the swelling in her legs gets worse* when she stands in one place for a long time without moving, and *instructions in some simple ankle exercises* she is to do whenever she is sitting or inactive to help pump the blood back up to her heart.

Mrs Dix has been an alert, cooperative patient who seems to have no difficulty remembering the instructions she has received and appears to be trying hard to follow them. However, she relies heavily on Cleo for reassurance and direction, and often apologizes for taking her time. Her conversations with Cleo often include such comments as, 'You must hate to see me coming', 'I don't know how I got into this mess', 'Was that all right?' and 'I don't know what I'd do without you.'

Today Mrs Dix arrived for her appointment 10 minutes late and somewhat out of breath. Her conference with Cleo began as follows:

Olive: *I'm sorry I'm late. I left work early and thought I had plenty of time, but the first five buses were full and went right by me without even slowing down. Five! Can you imagine! And of course there wasn't a cab in sight.*

Cleo: *Don't worry, I was a little behind schedule myself — and I know what buses are like this time of day. They really ought to put more drivers on. I can remember when you didn't have to wait — and when they didn't pack you in like sardines — and when the fare was only 15 cents!* (groans) *The good old days!*

Olive: Laughs. *You said it.*

Cleo: *Well, how's it been going?*

Olive: *Okay I guess. I've been trying to do everything you told me.*

Cleo: *Sticking to the diet?*

Olive: *Uh, huh.*

Cleo: *How about the stockings, have you been wearing them?*

Olive: *Yes, I've been a good girl.*

Cleo: *Great! Keep up the good work.*

At this point in their conversation, the clinic secretary came in, apologized for interrupting, and asked if Cleo could help her for just a minute with a question that had come in over the emergency phone. Cleo excused herself, dealt with the question, and started back to Mrs Dix. As Cleo passed her the secretary said, 'Thanks a lot. Say, how's Mrs Dix doing? Has she got her rubber suit on?' 'Rubber suit?' asked Cleo, 'What on earth do you mean?' 'Well,' replied the secretary 'last time she was here I heard her talking to another woman in the waiting room. She had a magazine with this ad for a rubber suit you could wear an hour a day that was guaranteed to make you lose ten pounds in a week. Mrs Dix said since she had to wear rubber stockings anyway, she might as well get one of the suits and lose weight too while she was at it. It sounded to me as if she was serious.' 'Great!' said Cleo and continued on to the examining room where Olive Dix was waiting.

As you think about this case, please assume the following:

• 10 minutes have now passed since Mrs Dix arrived. Cleo's next patient is due in 20 minutes.

• Prior to the conference Cleo decided that today she particularly wanted to help Mrs Dix work on the following objectives:

1. To become more accurate in predicting the effect specific activities may have on the swelling in her legs

2. To improve her ability to vary the foods she eats to include appropriate items other than those listed on the sample menus

3. To improve her self-concept by helping her overcome her feelings that she is physically unattractive and has no real control over what happens to her.

Then answer the following questions:

1. If you were Cleo Bryant, when you returned to your conference with Mrs Dix, what kinds of questions would you want to ask her in order to work on these three objectives? To answer please:
   - Choose one of the objectives
   - Plan at least two different questions related to it
     — The first of these should ask Mrs Dix to *report* on some aspect of her experience that you think may provide a good starting point for work on the objective—i.e. the question should make it likely she will report an event related to the objective
     — The second question should be a follow-up that asks Mrs Dix to try to *think about or react emotionally* to the event she reported in a way that will let her practice the behavior described in the objective you chose.
   Please *do not* write down things you would *tell* Mrs Dix. Write down examples of the *questions* you would ask. Because exact wording may be important, do write these questions out fully, don't just think about them.

2. If you could go back and start this conference over again from the beginning, would you do anything differently? Why?

3. What about the 'rubber suit'? Is this anything Cleo should take time for in the conference? If she does decide to discuss it, do you see any way she could have planned the sorts of questions she might ask about it *before* the conference began?

As with the other case exercises in this chapter, begin by answering these questions independently. Then, if you can, exchange your ideas with at least one other clinical teacher before you turn to the feedback section.

FEEDBACK ON EXERCISE 18

Question 1

A good way to begin your review of the questions you proposed for the rest of Mrs Dix's conference is to try to imagine how she might respond to each of them. Be as realistic as you can in this, and try to imagine several different ways she might answer. Then compare the type of thinking or valuing these answers represent with the behavior described in the objective you chose. Do they match?

If you are working with a group or partner, review each other's questions and expected answers by asking yourself:

- If I were Olive Dix, would I know what this question meant? Would I be able to tell what it is Cleo is asking me?

- How would I be likely to answer? Would I say any of the things my partner is expecting?

- If I did answer the second question as my partner expects, would this be because I had thought things through or reacted to them in the way the objective describes? Might I arrive at this answer by a very different process?

Thinking about these characteristics of your own or a partner's questions should help you decide whether they are clear and logically related to the objective.

You may also find it helpful to compare the wording of your questions with the samples in the following chart. Both thought processes and questions can be classified in several different ways, but this system should at least help you think about the relation between specific word choice and the type of response questions are likely to provoke.

FEEDBACK

SAMPLE QUESTIONS FOR DIFFERENT USES

Question type   **Sample wording**

Convergent — Questions with one best or 'right'
answer which ask the student to:

Recall   specific facts _____ Where is the _____? When did he
                                                      _____?

                  definitions _____ What is a _____?

                  standards _____ What is the normal value for _____?

                  procedures _____ How should you _____? Then what
                                                      should you do?

                  theories _____ Why does _____ usually result in
                                                      _____?

Construct   an answer by using information from
                  memory *or* from an outside reference to:

                  compare and contrast _____ Are these the same? Has it changed?

                  evaluate _____ Will that be enough? Is that a problem?

                  predict _____ What would happen if you? Will that make
                                                      a difference?

                  explain _____ Why do you think that happened?

                  apply and plan _____ How could you use _____ to do that?

                  generalize _____ How are these all similar?

Divergent —   Questions with many possible 'right'
                  answers that ask the student to:

Originate   ideas and suggest varied possibilities by

                  suggesting alternative explanations _____ What else might account for that?

                  predicting various outcomes _____ What other things might happen if
                                                            _____?

                  proposing different methods _____ Could you do that any other way?

Express values and reactions about

                  importance _____ Do you think that matters?

                  preference _____ Would you like to _____?

                  satisfactions _____ How did that feel?

                  goodness _____ Was that fair? Do you think it's wrong to
                                                      _____ ?

Objective 1 calls for skill in predicting. To help her practice this you will need to ask Mrs Dix to try to apply some general principle to help her forecast what will happen in a specific, future situation. The case tells you she already has learned some general principles about the way gravity and exercise may affect the circulation in her legs. You could ask her to apply these to specific things that have happened to her during the last several weeks. For example you could focus the discussion initially by asking her, 'Have there been any times during the last couple of weeks when the swelling in your ankles was bad?' (a reporting question) Follow-up questions to ask her to apply these principles to make predictions related to that particular event might be:

- Do you think it would have made any difference if you had. . . . .?

- Were you afraid that might happen—or was it a surprise?

- Is that likely to happen again if you. . . . .?

Objective 2 is a more complex goal than objective 1 because it really calls for two, very different, sorts of thought processes. To do what this objective describes, Mrs Dix must first use divergent thinking to originate new ideas for her meals, ideas that go beyond the samples provided to her earlier. Then, because it is important that these variations be appropriate as part of her diet, she must go on to use convergent thinking and evaluate the alternatives in terms of the guidelines she learned earlier. You may have emphasized only one of these in your question planning, but eventually both will be needed.

An example of some of the many questions that could ask her to practice this two step process might be:

- What did you have for supper last night? (reporting to establish focus)

- Can you think of anything different you might have had instead of the (names dish)? (divergent thinking to suggest alternatives)

- If you made that substitution, would your total calories for the day still be under——? (convergent thinking to evaluate)

Objective 3 is probably the most difficult of the three to plan for. It also has two different parts, since it describes two ways in which Mrs Dix' self-concept needs to be improved. It also uses a very general term 'self-concept', and then goes on to define this further only by stating two ways in which her present self-concept is poor. In order to do anything about this you would need to decide for yourself what positive type of thinking or feeling you think it would be best to substitute for these negative reactions. Your questions would then be designed to encourage Mrs Dix to practice the desirable behavior. For example, if you believe her anxiety about the appearance of her legs is the result of diffuse, unrealistic thinking, you might decide the best strategy would be to use questions to encourage her to test her fears against real events she may have been ignoring. In that case you might ask her:

- Was there any time this week you felt particularly embarrassed about the way your leg looked? (reporting)

- Did anyone say anything to you? For example, did anyone ask you how you hurt your leg? (comparing what actually happened with what she might have feared)

On the other hand, if you felt the best way to overcome her anxiety and feeling that she has no control over events would be to teach her to be more assertive, your questions might take a quite different direction. For example:

- Can you think of any time last week when you felt something you had to do at work made the swelling in your legs worse? (reporting)

- What would you like to do to change your work to try to keep that from being a problem? (originate a solution)

- Would you need to ask anyone if that was okay before you did it? (evaluate)

Choosing a questioning strategy is far too complex a process for us to discuss it usefully here. So far as this exercise is concerned, the important thing is that you have some logical reason for preferring the approach you took, and that your questions are selected and worded in such a way that they seem likely to elicit the kind of response you believe will be helpful.

Question 2

In the first few minutes of the conference reported in this case, Cleo Bryant did several things that may prove useful later in the discussion. Her initial chit-chat about the bus gave Mrs Dix time to settle down after her agitated arrival, and probably helped to set an informal, accepting tone that should make it easier for Mrs Dix to speak freely later. In her initial questions Cleo turned Mrs Dix' attention to her experiences during the preceding weeks, and began to focus the discussion on two areas of special concern. However, this is only a small first step towards active work on any specific objectives. Whatever her purpose, Cleo will need to find some way of moving towards a more definite and analytical review if she is to help Mrs Dix make productive use of the events she recollects. The very open-ended sort of questions Cleo used at first may be helpful in allowing the patient to steer the conference towards the things that concern her most (a move Cleo may especially want to encourage if one of her goals is to increase Olive's sense of control over the events in her life). However, so far this general fishing expedition seems to have netted very little.

Because the case instructions asked you to assume you had three quite specific objectives for this conference, you might have decided that if you were Cleo and could start this conference over again, you would start right out with questions that had a more specific reporting and analysis focus.

You might also have felt you would prefer to ask a series of increasingly specific questions on one topic (e.g. diet) before letting the discussion wander off to something else. Either a non-directive or a carefully focused beginning can be effective, so long as your plans for later parts of the discussion will allow both some chance for the patient to decide what to talk about and some opportunity for questions that encourage work on specific, valuable skills and attitudes. If the conference continues to wander along at its initial rather unanalytical level for the rest of the appointment, Mrs Dix is likely to be frustrated and will get little help with the problems that brought her in. On the other hand, if you structure the discussion too ruthlessly, you may shut off Mrs Dix's attempts to report significant events you could not have anticipated: events that could be good starting points for work on the objectives.

Time limitations are a major factor in planning. Half an hour isn't much time to work on three such different and important objectives. Some of the things you might have suggested changing in order to overcome this constraint are:

- Spend less time on friendly conversation at the beginning of the appointment so you can get down to business sooner

- Arrange with other staff not to be interrupted

- Schedule longer for the conference in the first place

- Help the patient learn to continue this analysis on her own by sharing at least the first two objectives with her, and suggesting a set of questions she can use to guide her thinking about events that occur during the next several weeks

- Concentrate most of the conference on only one of the three objectives so at least you can help Mrs Dix make useful progress in one area today—leave the others for later conferences.

Each of these might help you make better use of the conference, but each has both advantages and disadvantages. If you are working with other clinical teachers on this exercise, exchange ideas on whether you think the net result of any of these changes would be beneficial.

Time pressures create an additional concern when the teaching technique in use is questioning. The need to accomplish a great deal quickly may make the clinical teacher reluctant to allow students the thinking time they need to develop useful answers. Sadker and Sadker have criticized the 'rapid bombing rate' used by many classroom teachers in their questions of students.[3] They base their comments on several widely quoted studies by Rowe and Lake[4] which showed that the average amount of time classroom teachers allow students to answer a question is only one second. If the student(s) do not respond by the end of this very brief period, the teachers usually repeat the question, rephrase it, or call on another student. Rowe and Lake also studied the effect of increasing the wait time to from 3 to 5 seconds, and found that even this modest increase increased the length of the students' answers, made it more likely they would volunteer, increased the likelihood of appropriate answers and strengthened the students' confidence in their own answers, increased the proportion of inferences from evidence, and made students more likely to ask questions of their own. Who knows what might have happened if wait time had been increased to 10 seconds—or if the student had been asked a question and told to think about it for a day or week until he and the teacher met in conference again. Whatever changes you may have proposed for making efficient use of this short conference, they probably should be accompanied by a reminder to make a conscious effort not to rush the questioning process, and to allow the patient time to actually practice the types of thinking the conference is intended to help her learn.

Question 3

What, then, should Cleo do about the 'rubber suit' problem? Ignore it? Drop her original plan for questioning and substitute exploration of this issue instead? Or should she seek some way to incorporate that exploration into her work on the three designated objectives? This is only one quaint example of the many events that may create a diversion from the instructor's original plan for a conference. No one could hope to anticipate all the specific questions, problems, triumphs and information a student may encounter during the many hours he and the teacher are apart. Yet these events are not entirely impossible to consider in planning.

The first step towards planning is to think about broad categories of events that:

- are likely to occur spontaneously in one form or another as part of the student's independent activity, and

- have a clear enough relationship to one or more of our instructional objectives for that student to make us feel this type of event should not be ignored.

For example, we can reasonably expect that any patient who has such common problems as varicose veins, swelling of the legs and obesity is very likely to learn of something that seems like an attractive remedy from newspapers, magazines, radio, television, advertising, or the advice and experiences of family and friends. We can also expect that some of these remedies will be useful, but others may be worthless or dangerous for our patient. If one of our objectives is to teach the patient to make sensible judgments about future health care practices then, even though we cannot predict exactly when this will happen or what form the tempting remedy may take, we can begin to plan for incorporating it into our conference teaching.

The second step in planning is to think about how we can find out when one of these events has occurred. Usually the best way to do this is to plan questions that can be asked periodically during conferences that encourage reporting of the type of event about which we are concerned. For example, 'Sometimes you can get good tips from other people or from things you read. Have you run into anything lately that seemed as if it might be helpful to you?'

FEEDBACK

Finally, we can think about the types of questions we might use to help the student think about this event in a way we believe will be useful. Because we can't predict exactly what will happen, we can't plan these questions precisely, but we can decide on a general approach. For example, we can anticipate that sooner or later this patient will hear about some new 'easy' method of weight control, and we can decide in advance that when this happens we will want to use questions to encourage the patient to evaluate the method in terms of some of the general principles we have been teaching her. (For example, the principle that weight loss or gain depends on the balance between calories taken in and calories consumed.)

This will not eliminate all the surprises from conferences, but it helps the clinical teacher decide whether to ignore such an unscheduled event or to try to do something with it.

If your interest is primarily in staff education or fieldwork supervision, you may want to do this sort of 'contingency planning' for unscheduled but likely-to-occur events in the following categories:

- The trainee observes an experienced member of the staff performing a procedure in a way that seems very different from the way he was taught to do it.

- In the course of his unaccompanied clinical work the student has an encounter with a patient or staff member whose behavior is unreasonable, unpleasant or upsetting.

- The trainee experiences times when personal concerns or his own health problems interfere with his ability to do acceptable work.

By considering such events in our planning for conferences, we can do a great deal to make these dialogues truly relevant and productive for our students.

ROLE MODELS AND RELATIONSHIPS

Willard Waller once described schools as 'museums of virtue' where teachers struggle anxiously to provide stiff-necked models of flawless behavior for their students to respect and imitate.[5] Clinical teachers recognize the importance their behavior may have as a model for students, and in the clinic, as in the school, the model sometimes is musty and artificial. *Role modeling* may be little more than self-conscious enactment of a rigid list of behavioral commandments, representing a pattern of behavior few clinicians could manage to sustain amid the hurly-burly of normal practice. However, wisely used, role modeling can provide students with a useful image of practical ways in which abstract values can be translated into action in everyday practice.

Students are most likely to imitate the actions of a role model when the model's actions seem:

- *authentic* — not a pretense or something done primarily for the student's benefit,

- *relevant* — logically connected with the student's own present or future responsibilities, and

- *possible* — within the student's capabilities.

A virtuoso display of exotic skills may be admired, but it is less likely to provoke imitation by a student than a consistent pattern of simple, attractive actions the student can imagine performing himself. Differences in status between teacher and student sometimes make this difficult to achieve. For example, clinicians often seek help from other patients in modeling desirable behaviors to someone who has recently become severely disabled or disfigured. The model provided by one patient to another may be far easier to believe and imitate than a more technically correct performance by a healthy professional.

At its best, role modeling not only provides the student with examples of specific behaviors he can imitate, but helps him see the principles behind these actions. The significance of a role model's behavior lies principally in the values and attitudes his behavior reflects. Whether the role being modeled is that of patient or professional, it incorporates a set of social beliefs about goals and priorities, rights and responsibilities, what is important, what is good, and what is appropriate.

One of the clinical teacher's most complex tasks is to teach students a social role, to influence their adoption of the set of beliefs and expectations needed to play this part well. This attitudinal learning complements and influences mastery of the special knowledge and skills the role requires.

- The newly diagnosed diabetic patient who must prepare for a role in which a lifetime of special precautions about diet will be necessary must learn not only which foods to limit or avoid, but also learn to believe this is important enough to be worth the dissatisfactions it may involve.

- The student dietitian who is preparing to work with diabetic patients must learn not only that poor motivation may interfere with patients' compliance with a modified diet, but also to believe that it is her responsibility to help patients develop the attitudes compliance requires.

Such general attitudes and values may be expressed through any of a wide variety of specific actions, and the most useful method of expression often depends a great deal upon the particular situation at hand. Specific actions by a role model may come to have great symbolic value when they seem to students or instructors to represent the essence of an important belief. The instructor who prizes specific actions as key elements in the role she wants to portray must be careful, however, to keep these actions from developing a life of their own, and becoming mere ritual behavior. To establish a link between concrete actions and general beliefs, role modeling is often used in combination with *direct instruction*, with explicit discussion of values and the reasons for their significance.

Direct instruction on values also may take several different forms. Some of the most common are:

- *explicit directions to* the student to do or not do specific things, accompanied by an explanation of why this is important. (E.g., 'When you go up to the unit be sure to let the head nurse know you're there; no one likes to feel things are being done behind their back.')

- *comments on the student's actions*, analyzing the attitudes they appear to reflect and suggesting why this may be desirable or undesirable. (E.g., 'I liked the way you took time this morning to listen to Mr Mulloy's long story about the stock market. It showed you respect his need to be seen as a competent businessman. He must need that badly right now when he's not sure how well he'll recover from this stroke.')

- *comments on the instructor's own actions* with explanation of the reasons for this behavior. (E.g., 'I've got to recalculate these oxygen uptake values before I record them in Mrs Arvidson's chart, they look a little odd and I know Dr Bryant always pays attention to them when he's deciding about discharge.')

- *non-directive discussions* with students to help them clarify their own values and assess the pros and cons of different points of view. (E.g., 'If you tell Mary that what she does bothers you, how do you think she'll react?')

When role modeling and direct instruction are effectively combined they help students develop beliefs that are both strong and flexible, since on the one hand they are supported by concrete example and on the other by functional logic. This permits students to decide for themselves in a wide variety of situations when to imitate the specific actions of a mentor they admire and when to do something different.

Most clinical teachers are quite conscious of the efforts they make to use role modeling and direct instruction to help students learn desirable attitudes and values. They may be less aware of the influence they have through their *spoken and unspoken expectations*. We show other people what we think of them by what we expect of them. The instructor's expectations serve as a mirror for the student, and what he sees in that mirror may profoundly effect both his present self-concept and the kind of person he attempts to become. Our expectations thus may become self-fulfilling prophecies through the subtle but important influence they exert on student beliefs and behavior. In recent years this possibility has been explored by Robert Rosenthal and his co-workers in a series of controversial studies.[6] In experiments both with animals and with human subjects this research provides thought-provoking evidence that students whom the teacher expects to do well are more likely to succeed than those the teacher believes will do poorly—even when

achievement is measured objectively and all the students actually have equal ability.

Expectations may be equally powerful tools for teaching patients. Judith Miller and her associates have written with great practical insight of the many ways in which nurses can strengthen the self-concept of chronically ill patients and help them overcome feelings of powerlessness by expecting these patients to make simple yet significant decisions about their physical surroundings and daily schedule.[7]

The instructor's expectations may send the student a variety of significant messages:

- 'I believe you can do this job.'
- 'I expect you to be careless.'
- 'Your opinions are worth listening to.'
- 'You are a sensitive person.'
- 'I know you are trying hard.'
- 'You will never really be good at this.'

Such assessments and predictions may be communicated to the student in many different ways. For example, the instructor's view of the student's present performance and future potential may be reflected in:

- *the type and level of responsibilities* the student is assigned and the amount of supervision the instructor shows she thinks the student needs

- the instructor's *reactions to the student's suggestions* and willingness to take time to hear what the student has to say

- the *informal relationships* between instructors and students and whether they show the student is seen as a potential peer or as someone who cannot be fully trusted and has little to offer

- and, of course, in *direct statements* to the student about the instructor's perceptions of his talents, shortcomings and aspirations.

Particularly when student and teacher work together over a long period of time, their personal relationship may be a particularly important source of messages about the instructor's expectations. This is especially obvious in the styles adopted by different clinical supervisors during social interaction with professional students assigned to them for fieldwork experience. To some supervisors, a student is a student until the day he graduates, regardless of his level of technical and scientific competence. This view is reflected in a sometimes subtle, sometimes obvious social distance and witholding of regard for the student as a peer. To other supervisors, a student is a peer from the very beginning and treated socially as a professional colleague even though his mastery of important skills may still be very incomplete. Either pattern may send the student mixed messages about his current status, since in both there will be times when the supervisor's expectations of the student's competence do not match her belief that he should behave in a way that reflects acceptance of fully professional values and attitudes. This can create problems if it either discourages advanced level students from taking initiative and behaving as responsible peers, or if it gives students an unrealistically high, or low, opinion of their changing level of technical skill.

Role models, direct instruction and expec-tations are only a few of the many tools clinical teachers can use to shape and nurture the values and aspirations of their students. However, they provide useful examples of ways in which the attitudinal aspect of instruction can be planned and controlled to help students achieve instructional objectives in the affective domain. Use of these techniques of instruction calls for as much care and logic as those for helping students improve their judgmental skills and knowledge of scientific fact and theory. Planning begins with decisions about objectives—with clear identification of the values and attitudes that will be helpful to the student in the role for which he is preparing. The instructor then seeks ways to help the student find out what these values are, to let him actively experience them for himself, and to find satisfaction in this experience.

The following case will let you analyze a small sample of practical attempts to do these things.

INFLUENCING STUDENT ATTITUDES AND VALUES: THE CASE OF THE REALISTIC ROLE MODEL

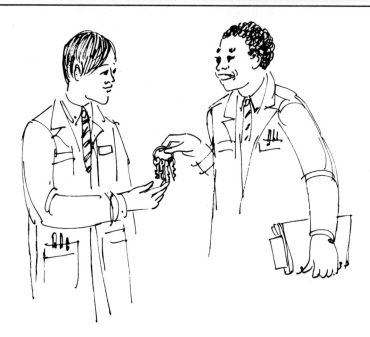

John Reed is a physical therapy student who will complete his professional education at the end of his current 6-week, full-time assignment to a 200 bed private rehabilitation center. He is now in the second week of this affiliation and is working under the supervision of Louis Duval, one of the center's senior staff therapists. On the first day of this assignment John and Louis spent nearly an hour talking about what this final piece of John's program should include. Because in an earlier affiliation at another hospital John had been mildly criticized for not having enough self-confidence, and for asking some of his patients to attempt things that were beyond their capabilities, he was anxious to improve in these areas. The list of nearly two dozen objectives John and his supervisor drafted during this meeting included the following two affective goals:

For John to develop:

1. commitment to thoroughness in evaluating individual patients' needs for and ability to tolerate specific types of treatment

2. confidence in his own ability to carry out professional tasks that require independent action and initiative.

In addition to providing treatment for the center's in-patients, this physical therapy department has an active out-patient service. Most of these treatments are given between 8:30 a.m. and 5:00 p.m. However, in order to accommodate patients who have full-time jobs, the department also schedules a limited number of early morning appointments. Staff take turns working an early schedule to treat these patients. An aide and one staff therapist are usually sufficient to do the work.

Yesterday morning, when John returned to the department office after attending a case conference, his supervisor said, 'John, I know we talked about having you spend most of your time this week up on the spinal injuries unit, but Linda, who's supposed to cover the early out-patients this week, just called in to say she has a bad case of flu and will probably be out for several days. I know you've had a good deal of out-patient experience, and you said you'd like to do some more work with low back pain patients. What do you think about shifting your schedule so you could take an early morning clinic? You could still spend the rest of the day on the spinal unit.' John responded, 'Sure, that's okay with me.' 'Great,' said Louis, 'That'll be a real help. I'll get together with you at 4 to go over the schedule and give you the keys.'

When they met at the end of the day, Louis showed John where the out-patient charts were kept and where he could find information on the treatment each of the four early morning patients scheduled for Tuesday was receiving. 'We try to keep this pretty detailed for these early patients, because the therapist on that shift changes quite often' Louis explained. He then told John about some of the mechanics of opening the clinic, recording the visits for billing and charting what he did. 'Edna, our most experienced aide, will be on with you.' He commented, 'She can help the patients get ready for treatment, and if you want her to she can give Mr Chavez his hot packs. The main reason we have her come in though is so you won't be alone if you need help, and to get the department ready for when most of the staff arrive. She's supposed to do things like put towels in the booths, fill the whirlpools if they'll be needed and make sure the weights are back on the cart. Edna knows what to do, but sometimes she skips things or does something like filling the whirlpool with hot water even though no one is scheduled to use it until two in the afternoon. Keep an eye on her would you?' 'You bet' said John. 'Okay. Here are the keys to the department. For god's sake don't lose them!' Louis cautioned him with a laugh. 'Go ahead and look over the charts. I'll be here for another 30 minutes. Let me know if you have any questions.'

John's work the next morning seemed to go smoothly, and when he met Louis in the staff room afterwards and was asked, 'How'd it go? Any problems?' John replied, 'No I don't think so. Do you want me to cover the early clinic again tomorrow?' 'Yes, if that's okay with you. There will be two back patients coming in you might like to see.' Then Louis added, 'Denise (another staff member) and I are just going to get a quick cup of coffee. Want to come along?' 'Sure', said John 'I'm not due on the spinal unit for another half-hour and breakfast was a long time ago.'

As they sat down at a table with their coffee, Louis asked Denise, 'You've been treating Mrs Brodsky haven't you?' 'Yes', said Denise. 'When I was up on her unit earlier this morning,' Louis explained, 'one of the nurses asked me if Mrs Brodsky couldn't have her crutches up in the room so they could encourage her to do more walking to build up her endurance. I said I'd check with you to see whether she's ready to walk alone yet. What do you think?' 'She knows what to do,' Denise answered, 'but when she starts talking to someone or gets to looking around, sometimes she forgets and puts too much weight on her bad leg.' 'Sounds to me as if you might want to hold off on sending her crutches up,' commented Louis, 'unless one of the nurses will have time to go with her any time she's walking. Will you get back to the nurse?' 'Yup. Gotta run. I've got a patient due' said Denise and hurried off.

Louis turned to John and said, 'You really have to be super cautious with some of these older orthopaedic patients. It just takes a couple of bad steps to really mess up a good piece of surgery. . . . Say, while we have a minute, tell me what you thought of Edna this morning. She's been here for 3 years, and she's good with the patients, but I'm worried because sometimes you just can't count on her to think about what she's doing.' 'She started out okay,' said John, 'I saw her charging around putting out the linens, and she did a nice job of putting Mr Chavez' hot packs on. But at about a quarter to 8 I noticed there was someone scheduled for the whirlpool at 8:30, and she hadn't filled it yet. I went into the staff room and she was reading the paper, so I asked her if there was anything I needed to do to get things ready for when the rest of the staff got there. She gave me kind of a blank look, but then she went over and checked the schedule, and went and filled the whirlpool. Maybe she needs to have a written list of things she's supposed to do each day. . . . but I guess that would just be one more thing for the staff to do wouldn't it?' 'Yes, it could be a nuisance,' responded Louis, 'but it might be something we could try as a last resort if this goes on being a problem. Anyway, I like the way you got her going. Nice move!' 'Thanks,' said John. 'Oh, by the way, Mr Chavez asked if next week he could come in on Wednesday morning instead of Tuesday. He has to be out of town Tuesday. I checked the schedule and it didn't seem too full so I told him that would be okay.' 'Oh boy,' groaned Louis, 'on Wednesday we always have a lot of last minute hurry-up appointments from hand clinic. That's why I explained to you last week we always have the secretary make all the appointments. She keeps track of all these things. I'll have to tell her to call Mr Chavez back and tell him Wednesday is no good.'

That afternoon, while John was up on the spinal unit and Louis was in the staff room making out charge slips for his patients, one of the orthopaedic residents stormed in. He said to Louis, 'Say, what have you been doing to Mr Nichols? He's supposed to be on a very gentle exercise program and when I went in to see him this morning his knee was swollen up like a balloon and he said it had been bothering him ever since he was down here yesterday afternoon.' 'That doesn't make sense,' said Louis, 'all I've been having him do is straight leg raising when he's here, and muscle setting 25 times an hour in his room. He does them both easily. We started with just the exercises here the first day and I checked when I was on his floor that afternoon to make sure he wasn't having any reaction. He knows he's not supposed to do anything else yet, and I've told him to stop if the muscle setting causes pain. I can't see why he's having problems.' 'Well all I know is that this is going to set him back at least a couple of days. You'll just have to be more careful!' said the surgeon and walked out. At this point another staff member who had been working in the staff room while this exchange took place, burst out, 'Who does that guy think he is? More careful! You did everything anyone could have to be careful!' 'Yeah,' sighed Louis,' 'well, at least I'm glad John wasn't here. I've been trying to get *him* to be more careful, and this sure wouldn't have been much help!' He paused, and then continued, 'I don't know though . . . maybe I ought to tell him about it. This sort of thing could happen to him. I'm not sure . . .'

Questions for review of the case

As with most other exercises in this book, you can analyze this case by yourself. However, to expand on the ideas presented in the feedback section you will find it valuable if you can arrange to discuss your responses to the following questions with at least one other clinical teacher.

1. At what points in the case description do you feel this supervisor did something that was probably *helpful* to John in achieving one or both of the two affective objectives? Especially if you will be exchanging your responses with someone else, go through the case and circle the sections that describe such helpful actions.

2. To which of the objectives is each of these helpful actions related?

3. How would you classify the technique the supervisor used at each of the points you marked?

   Was Louis:

   • giving John *direct instruction* about how he should think or feel, why this is important, or about how a specific action is related to some general value?

   • serving as a *model* to show John how the values in an objective might be implemented in actual practice?

   • or providing a *mirror* to help John see himself through his instructor's eyes and develop his own self-concept in response to the instructor's expectations?

4. Were there any points at which you feel the supervisor's actions were *unhelpful* or where Louis missed a good chance to do something that could have encouraged John to adopt the values in the objectives? If you had been the instructor, would you have done anything differently?

5. Finally, if you were the supervisor, where would you go from here? Would you continue to hope John never found out about your encounter with the surgeon, or would you plan to use this event to help him learn to cope with problems of this sort?

FEEDBACK

FEEDBACK ON EXERCISE 19

The supervisor in this case did several things that should help the student become more thorough and self-confident. He used both role modeling and direct instruction: For example:

- During the coffee break conversation with Denise, Louis provided a clear, practical *model* of the sort of careful assessment a thorough therapist might make as part of even a rather simple clinical decision (obj. 1). Louis did his 'checking' informally, quickly and with little fuss, but clearly showed he thought this was worthwhile—even though it interrupted a short break.

- He then followed up with an equally brief bit of *direct instruction* as he commented to John on how things can go wrong if you aren't careful in such cases (obj. 1 again).

However, Louis relied primarily on instructor *expectations* as a tool for encouraging John to feel confidence in his professional competence (objective 2).

- Throughout most of the activities described in the case, the supervisor's informal relationship with the student is that of a peer. Although Louis is still obviously 'in charge', such things as his invitation to John to come for coffee, the way he phrases his questions, and the time he took on John's first day at the center to involve him in selecting objectives all reflect his view of the student as someone whose opinion matters. Since John will graduate in only a few weeks, this seems more appropriate than an interaction style that says, 'You're not one of us yet—you're just a student.' This relationship provides a good background for the supervisor's more specific efforts to show John he sees him as capable of taking on assignments that call for independence and initiative.

- Louis demonstrates his confidence that John can function as a professional by asking him to fill in for another staff member, cover the early morning clinic without another therapist being present, and help in supervision and evaluation of a member of the support staff.

- Louis' treatment of John as a peer during their informal interactions extends into many of their discussions of professional matters. In reviewing patients for the early clinic, for example, Louis provides background information on the patients and on operating procedures in much the same way as he might do for a staff member who had not covered the clinic before.

- In his questioning of John about the aide's performance, Louis again shows his expectation that John may have useful information to offer and that his opinions are worth listening to. This is a very different kind of questioning from classroom quizzing of students to find out whether they know the right answer.

- This exchange is completed in a very positive way, with the supervisor admiring John's technique in reminding the aide to be thorough in completing her work (something that might help with both objectives 1 and 2). Louis is also careful not to simply dismiss John's ideas about how the aide could be reminded of her duties, even though it does not look like a winning solution to the problem. The instructor's expectations of competence are thus expressed in a variety of ways, and when competence is shown it is recognized and reinforced both by direct praise and by showing John's contributions have been useful.

However, the supervisor also did several things that conflicted with this generally positive message. You might feel these are useful since they help provide John with a realistic and balanced picture of his own still imperfect skills. On the other hand, you might be concerned about some of Louis' actions and feel he could provide realistic feedback in a more constructive way.

For example:

- Louis' comment about not losing the department keys, even if made in jest, hardly reflects confidence in John. Being given the keys might have considerable symbolic importance for the student, especially if he has never been given similar responsibility before. If so, Louis' 'joke' probably diminished the value this moment might have had for helping John achieve objective 2.

- His response to John's decision to reschedule a morning patient, while possibly quite justified in terms of departmental procedures, was expressed in an unhelpful way. John did make a mistake, and needs to know this, but by saying, 'I'll have to tell the secretary to call Mr Chavez' Louis seems to be telling John he doesn't have confidence in John's ability to correct his own errors. Instead of taking the matter entirely out of John's hands, Louis might have asked him to help decide whether a single therapist could handle Mr Chavez' treatment along with the other scheduled patients if several hand cases also showed up. Even simply asking John to arrange for the secretary to reschedule Mr Chavez would probably have been more positive. A small difference perhaps, but it is often through such undramatic exchanges that self-concept is developed. In any event this episode seemed to offer opportunities to help John learn to be thorough (obj. 1) that his supervisor failed to use to best advantage.

You may also have felt that had you been the supervisor you would have done additional things to use John's experience in the clinic to work on one or both objectives. For example, Louis made little attempt to talk with John about what should be covered in evaluation of any of the morning clinic patients either before or after John treated them, and the discussion of the aide's performance was superficial and stopped short of discussing whether their evaluation of her work was an adequate basis for planning supervisory action. Either topic could have been used for additional work on the two objectives. However, these goals must compete for attention with all the other important things John and Louis need to do. Since other opportunities for helping John develop self-confidence and commitment to thoroughness in evaluation are likely to come along later in his affiliation, you may have felt you would not want to spend more time on these objectives right now.

But what about the supervisor's own problems with his patient? How did you decide you would handle this?

The supervisor's initial relief that the student wasn't there to witness his frustrating exchange with the surgeon seems very natural. We often think of a role model as someone who shows the student how things ought to be done, a model of success. But this is only one side of the coin. The student also needs a model of how to behave when things go badly, a model of how to cope with failure.

This seems especially relevant for work on the two objectives at the center of this case. Professional practice in all health disciplines is filled with uncertainty. Even the most widely used and trusted methods of intervention and evaluation cannot be guaranteed to be effective and accurate. Too many unknown and unknowable factors may influence the individual patient's response for even an exceptionally competent clinician to feel confident that if he is skilled, thorough and caring he will also always be successful. Here then, Louis has a promising opportunity to model and discuss an appropriate response to this professional uncertainty and the 'undeserved' disasters it can create.

To make the most of this situation the supervisor would probably need to make use of a teaching technique that was not used during the activities described in the case summary — direct instruction through analysis of specific events. To do this the supervisor would need to set aside time to talk with John both about what happened in this particular situation, and about the sources of this sort of problem and some of the options for coping with it. Louis can model for

FEEDBACK

the student an honest and realistic approach to practice, but uncertainty is not a problem to which there is one clearly preferable response. Perhaps the best thing the supervisor can do is to allow enough opportunity for exploratory discussion of the issues for the student to recognize the importance of the problem and begin to consider his own solutions.

This sort of situation calls for a sturdy ego and a clear view of the principal objectives on the part of the supervisor. For example, Louis might be tempted to let the discussion shift into a condemnation of the resident's arrogance. Louis will need to decide which will be most valuable for the student, to learn how he might respond when a professional colleague is unfair or unpleasant, or to learn how to cope with the fact that despite his own thoroughness things went wrong. The patient's knee *is* swollen, and while Louis may or may not have caused this, he certainly did not expect it and must deal now with the results of an uncertainty even his skill and care could not eliminate.

This particular aspect of the case is perhaps most important as an example of the need to think long and hard about attitudinal objectives before attempting to model the values they involve. In this case it seems important to help John see both sides of self-confidence, and to recognize the limits of even expert thoroughness. In other situations quite different values may be at issue, but they too are likely to be multidimensional. Unless the clinical teacher gives careful thought to this complexity the model, instructions and expectations she uses to teach attitudes and values may be too simplistic to be of real value.

NOTES TO CHAPTER 4

1. Ausubel D 1963 The psychology of meaningful verbal learning. Grune & Stratton, New York
2. Kadushin A 1976 Supervision in social work. Columbia University Press, New York, pp 166–167
3. Sadker M, Sadker D 1977 Questioning skills. In Cooker J M (ed): Classroom teaching skills: a handbook. D.C. Heath, Lexington, Mass
4. Rowe M 1973 Teaching science of continuous inquiry, pp. 243–73, McGraw-Hill, Lake J H 1973 The influence of wait-time on the verbal dimension of student inquiry behaviour. Doctoral Dissertation, Rutgers University
5. Waller W 1932 The sociology of teaching. John Wiley, New York
6. Rosenthal R, Jackson L 1968 Pygmalion in the classroom: teacher expectations and pupil's intellectual development Holt. New York
7. Miller J 1983 Coping with chronic illness: overcoming powerlessness. F. Davis, Philadelphia

5 USING EVALUATION AS A TEACHING TOOL

FORMS AND FUNCTIONS OF EVALUATION

To some teachers evaluation means telling students when they make mistakes and giving them grades; to others it means keeping track of how students are progressing and letting them know what they are doing right. Evaluation is all these things—and much more. It is a process that uses many different methods and serves many different purposes. To understand the reasons for these differences and see how the format of an evaluation is influenced by its purpose it is helpful to classify some of the types of evaluation clinical teachers use most often, using the two categories suggested by Benjamin Bloom.[1]

1. *Formative evaluations* that monitor student performance at frequent intervals and provide the detailed, diagnostic information needed for:

   - *feedback* to students about the specific strengths and weaknesses of their current performance

   - *planning* for future instructional activities

   - *individualization* of instruction to match the student's personal abilities, interests, style and level of achievement.

2. *Summative evaluations* carried out at the end of a major block of instruction to provide the condensed, overall picture of student achievement needed for:

   - 'gatekeeping' decisions concerning whether the student has mastered essential skills at the level necessary for safe, effective, independent performance

   - *recognition* of superior performance that should be rewarded by something such as a raise, promotion, honor, praise or special privilege

   - *record keeping and communication* to others (e.g., other supervisors, other health professionals involved in a patient's care) concerning the types and levels of skills the student has learned

   - *accountability* on the part of instructors and instructional programs for teaching effectiveness, efficiency and relevance.

STEPS IN THE PROCESS

While formative and summative evaluations differ in many obvious ways they also have much in common. Both types of evaluation make use of a process that includes the following basic steps:

1. Choosing a *focus*—deciding exactly what it is we want to evaluate

2. Planning a *method of measurement*—deciding which observable features of the performance to use as the basis for our evaluation and how we will collect information on them

3. Setting a *standard*—specifying the degree to which the measured features of performance must be present in order for students' learning to be judged acceptable

4. Collecting *data*—by carrying out the measurements we have planned on a sample of the work of a real student

5. Making a *judgement*—to decide how the measured characteristics of the real performance compare with those in the standard we established earlier

6. *Communicating* the results of our evaluation to the student and to others concerned in his instruction.

The exercises in this chapter provide you with opportunities to practice these steps within the context of some of the evaluative tasks clinical teachers undertake most frequently. They emphasize formative evaluations based on observed performance of realistic tasks.

DECIDING WHAT TO EVALUATE

When we evaluate learning we evaluate the degree to which our instructional objectives have been achieved. If these have been clearly formulated they will tell us what sorts of specific, useful tasks our students should be able to perform if our teaching, and their learning, are successful. Chapter 2 of this Handbook includes several exercises concerned with methods for selecting and describing objectives. The bibliography for that chapter suggests a number of excellent sources of additional help on this important step. If you do not feel confident of your ability to set behavioral objectives you may want to do some preparatory work on this skill now, since it is the foundation for all the other steps in the evaluation process. This review also will

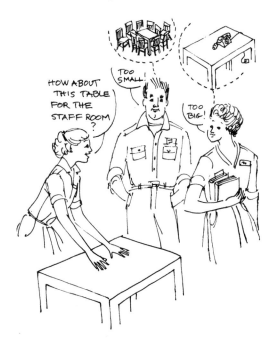

HOW ABOUT THIS TABLE FOR THE STAFF ROOM?

TOO SMALL!

TOO BIG!

remind you of a general guideline of particular importance for formative evaluation: the most useful evaluations of learning judge the student's demonstrated ability to perform well-defined, useful tasks rather than his apparent possession of general personal or professional traits. Such characteristics as trustworthiness, initiative, problem-solving ability and creativity are important; but they are too diffuse and ambiguous to evaluate fairly unless they are linked to some of the specific tasks for which they are needed.

DECIDING HOW TO MEASURE LEARNING AND WHAT STANDARD TO USE FOR JUDGING RESULTS

To evaluate learning the teacher samples what the student is able to do and draws more general conclusions about mastery from these measurements. The first step is to decide what aspects of the student's work to consider. We need to select factors that are both easy to observe and convincing as evidence of the particular type of learning we want to assess. Unlike the classroom teacher, who often must rely heavily on paper and pencil tests or performance under simulated conditions, the clinical teacher usually can judge what the student has learned by seeing how he performs practical tasks in a realistic setting. This realism helps make our evaluations valid, but it is not without its hazards. Real clinical work often is both private and complex. The student's performance may be awkward to observe, and when several different skills are used in combination they may be difficult to tease apart and evaluate separately. Sometimes we focus our attention on how the student goes about performing a learned task, at others we judge his learning primarily by looking at the results he gets. Whichever we choose, we must ask ourselves, 'Will this really tell me whether the student has learned what is necessary?'

As thinking about evaluation progresses it becomes more and more specific. In addition to deciding what types of action we will use as indices of learning, we also must consider:

- what qualities to take into account in deciding whether each component is correct

- under what conditions we want the student to be able to perform

- how often we need to see a student attempt the task before we feel prepared to judge his level of mastery

- what types or degrees of error would make us say mastery is not yet acceptable.

For example, deciding to judge whether a student has learned to take blood pressure readings by looking at the way she handles the equipment and by comparing the results she gets with our own is only a partial plan for evaluation.

We still must answer such questions as:

- Should we consider only whether she goes through all the required steps in the procedure in the correct order—or also take into account the speed and smoothness with which she does this?

- How closely must her readings match ours to be acceptable?

- Will we be satisfied if she can do the procedure correctly in a quiet area with a cooperative patient whom she knows well—or must she be able to perform in an area full of interruptions and distractions or with patients who are unfamiliar or uncooperative?

- If she does this correctly once will that be enough to convince us she has learned what is necessary, or do we need to see a number of attempts to make a judgment?

The literature on educational evaluation is filled with useful suggestions on how to deal with such questions. In designing valid, reliable and practical methods of evaluation however, clinical teachers have another valuable source of help— each other. This is an area of teaching in which exchanging ideas with colleagues is of special value. Exercise 20 will let you practice using a special group process to decide how to evaluate one type of learning.

DRAFTING CRITERIA FOR RATING A CLINICAL SKILL

In this exercise you will work with a small group of other clinical teachers to make up a list of specific criteria you could use to judge a student's mastery of one type of skill. Since the method you use is designed to let you take advantage of other people's ideas, the exercise will be most useful if you do it with four or five others. If this is impossible, you can do the work with just one partner.

Allow at least 1 hour to complete all tasks. If you wish, Tasks A,B,C and D may be done on one day and E, F and G on another.

TASK A Form a work group

To allow everyone to take an active part in discussion, limit the group to not more than six members. Several groups can do the exercise at once.

If possible, work with other clinical teachers whose work situation and teaching responsibilities are similar to your own. This will make it easier for you to select the skill to be rated and to think realistically about the situation in which your ratings might be done.

TASK B Decide on the focus of your evaluation

Begin by deciding what sort of *student* you want to evaluate, and in what type of *situation* you will imagine you are observing his performance. Write a summary of what you decide in the spaces at the top of the attached worksheet.

Then select the *type of learning*—the clinical skill—you want to evaluate. You may choose one from the following list of examples or propose one of your own. The skill you choose should be one with which all members of the group feel familiar, and be something that is complex enough so a correct performance involves several different factors.

Suggested skills

If you are planning to evaluate a fieldwork student or staff trainee, you might select a skill such as:

1. Ability to use good body mechanics when handling equipment and assisting patients

2. Ability to establish priorities among the components of a plan of care designed to achieve several different physical and psychosocial goals

3. Ability to write accurate and useful reports of his/her patient's problem, treatment and progress for inclusion in the medical record

4. Ability to cope with his/her own emotional reactions when the behavior of a patient with whom he/she is working becomes frightening, embarrassing, frustrating or otherwise upsetting.

If you are planning how to evaluate a patient or family member's learning, consider such skills as:

1. Ability to accurately perform a specific test related to their own health status (e.g. blood pressure, breast self-examination, urine testing)

2. Ability to carry out a recommended therapeutic or preventive regimen at home (e.g. select and prepare foods for a nutritionally balanced low cholesterol diet, do a graded series of strengthening exercises, or take a prescribed medication as directed)

3. Ability to assist or give recommended care to a family member or friend (e.g. communicate effectively with a deaf child using a sign language, encourage and support a recent stroke patient's efforts to feed and dress himself, give chest percussion and vibration during postural drainage to a person with bronchiectasis).

TASK C Orient yourself to the process you will use

The work you do during this exercise will be divided into three different stages:

- individual work to generate ideas for possible criteria

- uncritical pooling of suggestions from all group members

- critical review and revision of suggestions to select a master list the whole group can accept.

Based on a group process developed by Delbeque, this combination of individual and collective work is designed to encourage all members of the group to contribute their ideas before any critical discussion begins.[2] This recognizes that some people find it difficult to speak in a group even if they have good ideas, and if their initial suggestions are ignored or criticized this may discourage further participation. The final stage of the process recognizes that group members can help each other clarify their ideas and overcome personal biases by questioning suggestions they don't understand or that seem unimportant. To take full advantage of this process please follow the instructions for each step closely.

TASK D Work independently to make a list of your own ideas on how to evaluate this skill (allow at least 15 minutes for this step)

Without discussing your ideas, make a written list of specific things you would want to see a student do in order to feel convinced he had learned this skill at an acceptable level.

Set a standard for the performance based on what the student needs to do to be safe and effective on his own when your teaching is completed. Don't think in terms of some less adequate level of performance that might show encouraging progress at an early stage in instruction.

Try to choose aspects of performance that are:

- *Observable*—things you can see, hear or feel someone do or features of the end results of action that are easy to see

- *essential*—not simply desirable, or characteristics of an excellent performance, but *necessary* in order to be acceptably safe, effective and/or efficient

- *directly related to this skill* rather than primarily part of a different type of skill that may be used concurrently

- *likely to be called* for under most circumstances when this skill is employed rather than an aspect of performance needed only in really unusual situations.

Describe each aspect of performance you list as clearly as possible, using words others will find easy to interpret. A sample set of criteria for rating skill in infection control is attached to give you ideas for format and wording.

TASK E Share individual lists of criteria (allow about 10 minutes for this. If there are more than four people in your group you probably will need longer)

Select one member of your group to be recorder.

Go around the group taking turns reading out your criteria. Each person should read only *one* criterion each time it is his turn. Do *not* let anyone read their entire list at one time.

Have the recorder write down each criterion exactly as it is given. Do not reword or combine even if criteria seem quite similar. Use a blackboard or large piece of paper. Criteria should be written large enough for all group members to be able to read.

Do *not* begin to comment on any of the criteria yet. The purpose of this step is to get *all* ideas down.

If you get new ideas for your own list from something another person says you may add them.

Continue this until each member of your group has read *all* the things they listed. Even if some appear to duplicate others already read by someone else they should be mentioned. If the wording suggested by two people is completely identical the recorder may simply put a mark in front of the statement to show it was suggested twice—but if they are somewhat different write both down.

Remember—do not criticize, discuss, reword, combine or omit anything at this stage. Just get it all down.

TASK F Discuss, revise and select a master list of criteria (25 minutes)

Select one member of your group to be the discussion leader.

Now discuss and revise your collection of suggested criteria. Your purpose is to reduce them to a list of not more than 10 clear descriptions of things anyone performing this task must do in order for his performance to be judged acceptable. Consider each of the following questions:

1. Are some suggestions *worded unclearly?* If so, revise them until all members of the group feel they know what the statement means. If you can't accomplish this, discard the suggestion.

2. Do some suggestions *duplicate* each other? If so, try to combine them in a way that does justice to all versions of the idea.

3. Are any *not* stated in terms of an *observable* action? If so, try to reword them into descriptions of actions someone other than the performer could see, hear or feel.

4. Are any *impractical* to rely on because they are only called for under special circumstances or are unlikely to be exhibited when another person is observing? If so, discard.

5. Are any really *unnecessary* as part of an 'acceptable' performance? Discard any that are desirable but not absolutely essential.

6. Are any of the criteria really *not directly related* to the specific skill your group is considering? If they primarily concern a different skill omit them—even if they are important for *overall* competence as the type of professional or patient you are considering.

7. Finally, do the remaining criteria provide you with a list that is *complete* enough to let your group feel 'if someone did all these things we would be confident their skill was acceptable'? Remember, you do not have to list everything that matters so long as the criteria you do list seem adequate to screen out incompetence.

As you make the changes and additions agreed to by the group the recorder should write these on the master list.

TASK G **Make a legible copy of your master list**

By now your working list is probably quite messy. Make a clean copy on one of the attached forms using ink or very dark pencil so you can photocopy it for each member of the group.

As you do this take a few minutes to think about the order in which the criteria should be listed. Sometimes it is best to list them in the sequence in which they are likely to occur, but for other skills grouping-related criteria may make them easier to use.

SAMPLE* The following sample shows a useful level of detail for criteria.

CLINICAL SKILL RATING SHEET

Type of student: *Fieldwork student on clinical assignment or newly employed staff member.*

Setting: *Medical or surgical in-patient unit of a general, acute-care hospital.*

Skill: *Ability to follow institutionally approved procedures for infection control.*

Rating		Performance criteria
OK	not OK	1. *Washes hands thoroughly according to instructions in the hospital's procedure manual before and after each patient contact and/or before handling supplies.*
OK	not OK	2. *Keeps 'dirty' items separate from 'clean' items and areas.*
OK	not OK	3. *Disposes of contaminated dressings and supplies according to the hospital's policies.*
OK	not OK	4. *Handles sterile instruments and supplies only with sterile forceps or sterile gloves.*
OK	not OK	5. *Allows only sterile instruments and supplies to contact patient's wound site or surgical incision.*
OK	not OK	6. *Uses protective clothing (cap, gown, mask) to reduce airborne contamination to patient or self when called for by institutional procedure manual.*
OK	not OK	7. *Follows the hospital's infection control procedures in transporting and assisting patients who require special handling to control spread of infection (either to or from the patient).*
OK	not OK	8. *Recognizes when inadvertent contamination of sterile or clean objects and areas has occurred and takes corrective action consistent with institutional procedures.*

Anecdotal notes on significant observations and comments on other aspects of performance that are important indicators of acceptable mastery or deficiencies in mastery:

* Based on a rating sheet from *The Blue Macs, Mastery and Assessment of Clinical Skills* developed by the Texas Consortium for Physical Therapy Clinical Education.

EXERCISE 20

CLINICAL SKILL RATING SHEET

Type of student:

Setting:

Skill:

Rating		**Performance criteria**: Key indicators of acceptable mastery
OK	not OK	1.
OK	not OK	2.
OK	not OK	3.
OK	not OK	4.
OK	not OK	5.
OK	not OK	6.
OK	not OK	7.
OK	not OK	8.
OK	not OK	9.
OK	not OK	10.

Note: Each criterion will be rated *OK* if done acceptably or *not OK* if it is done incorrectly or not at all.

FEEDBACK ON EXERCISE 20

Perhaps the best way to get feedback on your rating criteria is to try using them in a real clinical situation. To do this:

A. Make several copies of the master list of criteria your group developed and wrote on the *Clinical Skill Rating Sheet* form.

B. Find at least one professional colleague who did *not* help to develop the criteria and who is willing to use the rating sheet to evaluate several students you both will have an opportunity to observe.

C. After you have both had time to use the criteria to evaluate several students, arrange to discuss the following questions:

1. Were the criteria *practical* to use as a basis for your evaluation?

   • Did you have a chance to see the students do these things?

   • Were you able to do this without disrupting your own schedule or interfering with the student's work and interaction with others?

2. Did your ratings seem *reliable*?

   • When you and your co-worker both evaluated the same student, did you agree on your ratings for each criterion?

   • Did each of you feel you were able to be quite consistent in deciding when to rate a criterion action *OK* or *not OK*?

3. Did you feel your evaluations were *valid*?

   • Did your co-worker agree that each of the criteria was important in deciding whether the performance was acceptable?

   • Did he or she think all the criteria were easy to understand?

   • How confident did you feel that the student's overall mastery of this skill was acceptable if you rated all the criterion actions *OK*? Did you still have doubts about the skill of any students who did all the things on your list acceptably? Did you ever feel certain a student really had mastered the skill even though they were rated *not OK* on some of your criteria?

4. Would the results of this evaluation be *useful* to you in making practical decisions about this student?

   • Did you both feel the standards set here were reasonable as a basis for deciding whether the student is ready to use this skill without assistance and supervision?

   • Could you use this list to help you pick out specific weak points in performance and plan your follow-up teaching to overcome them?

A second excellent way to get feedback on your work is to share copies of your criteria with several of your students. Choose students who match the description at the top of your skill sheet and who are now in the process of learning this particular skill. Ask them to use the criteria to assess their own performance for several days when you can arrange to observe and rate them too. Then discuss the following questions:

1. Does this list of criteria seem *fair*?

   - Do all of the actions listed really seem necessary?

   - Is it easy to judge whether another person is doing each of these things correctly, or does that seem to be mostly a matter of personal opinion?

   - If the student usually does these things correctly will the supervisor have a chance to see this?

2. Does the list seem *useful* to the student?

   - Did he or she feel fairly confident using the list to evaluate his/her own performance?

   - Did it help him/her know what was expected and make it easier to do the right things?

   - If the overall performance was still not acceptable, did the list of specific ratings make it easier to understand what the problem was and to plan how to correct it?

3. Did you and the students *agree* on your ratings?

Don't feel you must change everything another person says they find confusing, unrealistic or unnecessary; but if these comments are repeated they should help you see where additions, deletions or rewording are needed.

Alternative feedback method

If you did Exercise 20 as part of a clinical teaching course or workshop that included enough people so there were several different groups each working on their own set of rating criteria, you may find it helpful to exchange lists with another group. Give each member of the other group a copy of your master list and allow time for careful reading. Then review with the other group their reactions to the list of seven questions you used to help you select and revise criteria when you did Task F in the exercise. Their fresh point of view may help you find problems, and if they are positive in their reaction this should reassure you that the criteria would be useful even if used by a clinical teacher who had no part in their development.

IMPROVING THE QUALITY OF OBSERVATIONAL RATINGS

Clearly stated objectives and rating criteria take much of the guesswork out of student evaluation, but often they cannot stand alone. Rater training may be needed to prepare teachers to apply these guidelines appropriately. When the learning to be evaluated is simple and highly standardized, such rater training may be unnecessary. The correct performance can be described in a detailed, step-by-step list of necessary actions that requires little practice to interpret and use. However, much clinical learning is not that simple. Particularly when we consider the many complex judgmental and communication skills professional staff and students are expected to master, the following problems are obvious:

- There is often more than one right way to do things and the best way to do some things often depends on the specific situation. What is appropriate under one set of circumstances may be quite unacceptable under others. Evaluating performance of such a skill using a single set of rigid criteria is unreasonable.

- Opportunities for observation of the student's performance often are rushed and fragmentary. The supervisor cannot be with the student all of the time and important aspects of his work may go unobserved. Most judgmental steps cannot be observed directly. The supervisor must guess at the student's overall mastery on the basis of the bits and pieces of performance he can see, and often must rely heavily on what the student reports he does rather than on first hand observation.

- Finally, when the supervisor does have a chance to watch the student at work, the student frequently does several different things at once, using a variety of learned skills to carry out a single complex clinical job. The instructor must try to keep track of all this—usually without any opportunity to make notes during the observation—and then must analyze it to think about the different types of learning involved so the student's progress in each component can be evaluated separately.

Applying even a very good set of rating criteria can be difficult under such circumstances. Substantial practice and critical feedback from other teachers may be needed to prevent personal bias, confusion and oversight from damaging the validity and reliability with which criteria are applied.

Exercise 21 describes one technique clinical teachers can use for helping each other sharpen their rating skills.

RATING AN OBSERVED PERFORMANCE

In this exercise you will practice applying a set of rating criteria to evaluate a performance simulated through role playing. This will serve two purposes:

- to let you practice making some of the complex judgments such evaluations require, and

- to allow you to practice critiqueing a set of rating criteria by seeing how adequate they are when put to use.

This exercise must be done with a group.
Please allow from 45 minutes to an hour to complete all the tasks.

TASK A **Form a work group**

You will need to work with at least three other people to complete this exercise. It may, however, be done by a much larger group if you wish, so long as you have a room with a raised stage or open area so that everyone can see and hear what goes on during the role playing segment.

If your group is small, the exercise will be easiest to do if all participants are from the same professional field and have had some experience working in similar health care settings.

TASK B **Familiarize yourselves with the rating form and exercise instructions**

The performance you evaluate during this exercise will be an interview of a patient or family member by a health professional.

The criteria you will use for evaluating the simulated performance are listed on the rating form attached to these instructions. Read the rest of the instructions for the exercise to see what is expected and then look carefully at the criteria. *Do not* discuss them at this point even if you feel they are incomplete, unclear in places, or that some criteria might not be accepted by many people in your field. You will have an opportunity to critique and revise the criteria when you do Task H later in this exercise.

TASK C **Select two members of your group to do the role playing**

One group member should take the part of a fieldwork student or staff trainee who will carry out the interview. This is the person whose performance the other group members will evaluate.

The second person will take the part of a patient or family member, the 'client' who is being interviewed.

TASK D **Prepare for the role playing segment**

If you are one of the people who has agreed to take a part in the role playing, meet with your partner to do the following:

- Define the two characters you will play. Who are the two people involved and what is their relationship?
- Decide in what setting the interview will take place.
- Agree on the purpose of the interview.
- Discuss briefly anything you particularly want either of the two characters to do during the performance.

This planning does not need to be elaborate—just enough to let you, and your audience, imagine that this is a real performance. For example, you might agree on something as simple as the following.

This person doing the interview is a senior physical therapy student who is talking with a 45-year-old city bus driver whom he has been treating twice weekly for low back pain for the last month. The interview takes place in a treatment cubicle in the out-patient unit of a community hospital; and its purpose is to find out whether there has been any change in the patient's pains during the 3 days since the last visit and what the patient's activity level has been.

Please use the term 'interview' in its broadest sense to mean any series of questions asked by a health professional (or student) to get information from a patient or a member of the patient's family. This might be a formal interview such as a history, or might be the sort of questioning described in the preceding example.

To allow the other participants time to evaluate your performance, please plan a type of interview that will take at least 4 or 5 minutes to complete. We will allow a maximum of 15 minutes for the role playing part of this exercise. If the interview you plan is one that ordinarily would take longer than this, please role play the beginning of the interview and continue for about 15 minutes. At that point we will ask the raters to assume they have been called away before the interview is completed and must base their evaluation on the part they observed.

Try to make both characters seem as natural as possible. You can decide for yourselves how good a job the staff member/student will do—either doing the best interview you can, or building in some of the errors you think a person might make if they had not yet fully mastered this skill. The patient also can decide how cooperative, talkative, etc. he or she will be. However, you should try *not* to have either character do anything so outrageous that it makes realistic practice of evaluation difficult for the other participants.

If you are one of the participants who will be evaluating the simulated performance, take a few minutes to help make any physical changes in the room needed to clear a place for the role playing and arrange seating so all of you can see and hear what takes place. Then use the rest of the time to study the rating criteria and rating key. You will need to think about these as you watch the role playing and should have them clearly in mind before it begins.

TASK E **Present and rate the simulated performance**

The role players should begin by explaining to the group who each of them will pretend to be, the purpose of the interview, and in what sort of setting to imagine it is taking place.

The other participants should observe without interrupting or comment.

One group member should take responsibility for keeping track of the time. Please allow a maximum of 15 minutes for the role playing. Then, even if the interview is still not completed, ask the group to imagine they have been called away to do something else and will not be able to see the rest of the interview. Evaluations will be based on the part of the interview that was observed.

TASK F **Record your evaluations**

Use the attached rating form to do this.

Assign one of the following ratings for each of the specific criteria, and then summarize them to assign an overall rating for each of the three general aspects of performance (A, B and C).

Excellent	— This aspect of the performance was without error and included something that was unusually valuable and reflected a high level of skill.
Acceptable	— The interviewer did this consistently enough to make the questioning useful and acceptable to the patient even if there were some minor errors or omissions.
Unacceptable	— The interviewer failed to do this consistently, or attempts to do it were so flawed this significantly interfered with the usefulness of the questioning or was upsetting to the client.
Uncertain	— The part of performance observed provided too little activity related to this criterion to assign it a rating.

As you do this, please make notes on a separate piece of paper of any specific actions (or failures to act) by the interviewer that you felt were especially important in assigning a rating. If you noticed the interviewer do (or fail to do) something you felt was significant that was not directly related to one of the criteria on the rating sheet, make a note of this, too.

TASK G **Tabulate the ratings given by the group**

With one person serving as recorder, write down the number of people who gave each rating for each of the criteria. If your group is small you can probably do this on one of the rating forms. If there are more than five or six participants, put the tally on a blackboard or flip chart so every one can see the distribution.

TASK H **Analyze and discuss your tabulations**

Review the summary of ratings for each criterion giving special attention to the following questions:

1. *Are you satisfied with the level of agreement* (objectivity or inter-rater reliability) on ratings? Think about this in practical rather than statistical terms? If this were a real student or staff member being rated by several different supervisors, is it likely that one might say the performance was acceptable while another said it was not? Was there a clear pattern of agreement among most participants on what the rating should be even if one or two people disagreed?

2. *If you found considerable disagreement on any criterion can you explain why this happened?* Ask someone who gave a low rating and someone else who gave a high one to explain why they evaluated the performance as they did? Discuss the comments individual raters wrote describing specific incidents that influenced them. See if you think any of the following might have contributed to differences in ratings:

   • Some raters noticed things others overlooked.

   • Some took into account actions that others felt weren't directly related to the particular criterion being rated.

- Raters differed in the importance they attached to specific actions.

- The standard used to decide what was acceptable and what was not differed from rater to rater.

3. *Can you suggest changes that are needed* in the rating scale and general instructions or in the wording of the criteria in order to clarify points that are ambiguous?

4. *Did the group notice aspects* of the interviewer's performance *that seem important but are not covered* by any of the criteria? Does this justify adding any new criteria?

5. *Do any of the criteria seem irrelevant or unnecessary* for evaluating this particular skill? Should any be deleted or reworded?

6. *Did many raters give an uncertain rating* for some criteria? Would this be likely to occur in a real clinical setting also, or was it simply because the simulation was so brief or seemed artificial? If some participants felt unable to rate a particular criterion but others did not, what accounted for this difference? Can you suggest ways in which the criteria could be modified to make it more practical to gather information on important aspects of performance?

7. *Did you find any practical problems* in using the rating form? Would it be easy to use in a real clinical setting—epecially if this were only one of a variety of different clinical skills you needed to evaluate?

TASK I **Repeat the rating process with a new simulation**

Either now or at an early date, ask two other members of your group to role play a different interview. As you compare ratings on this performance give special attention to whether the earlier practice and discussion along with any change you made in the criteria helped to increase your level of agreement and your confidence in doing the evaluation.

Even if you have not made any major changes in the list of rating criteria on instructions for rating, the discussion of reason for difference in opinion should have brought your group members closer together in their interpretation and application of the evaluation criteria. The very best of evaluation forms often include some points that are confusing until they are discussed. For this reason, practice sessions such as this may be needed every now and then to help a group of staff who share responsibility for supervising the same students evaluate those students accurately and consistently.

OBSERVATIONAL RATING FORM

Skill evaluated: Carries out effective formal and informal interviews of clients to gain information needed for planning or evaluation of care.

Rating Criteria	Rating
A. Makes a well-organized attempt to secure all pertinent information.	_____overall
• Asks questions on all important topics at an appropriate level of detail	_____
• Restates client response when necessary to clarify or summarize meaning	_____
• Follows a logical progression without seeming inflexible	_____
• Completes the interview in a reasonable time	_____
B. Uses effective verbal communication.	_____ overall
• Expresses questions in simple and unambiguous sentences using terms the client understands.	_____
• Avoids 'leading' questions and restatement of responses that 'put words in the client's mouth'	_____
• Speaks audibly and without irritating verbal mannerisms	_____
• Interprets the client's verbal responses accurately.	_____
C. Establishes and maintains good rapport with the client throughout the interview.	_____ overall
• Begins the conversation by putting the client at ease	_____
• Uses body posture, eye contact and gestures that suggest attentiveness, approachability, and acceptance	_____
• Acknowledges and shows acceptance of client responses	_____
• Allows the patient time to answer throughtfully and to ask questions of his/her own.	_____

Notes

EXERCISE 21

FEEDBACK ON EXERCISE 21

Your best source of feedback on this exercise is the discussion of ratings and criteria you did during Task H. If you missed important observations, were biased in your interpretations, let your judgments be influenced by factors that really aren't directly related to the skill you evaluated, or if your personal standards were unrealistic, the ratings and comments of the other members of your group should have helped you discover and correct these errors.

As you reflect on these discussions, here are some more general recommendations to consider.

1. Remember, the majority isn't always right. Just because some of your ratings were different from those of most other group members doesn't automatically mean you were wrong. However, such differences should make you stop and think why you rate as you do. If you find you can't give a logical reason for your ratings, or that you consistently rate higher or lower than most other people, you should take time soon to analyze your own rating logic critically.

2. Take the circumstances of performance into account. One obvious reason why you might disagree with other clinical teachers on the ratings you give is that different work situations may call for a very different standard of skill in performing common tasks. For example, if one member of your group works in a home care program and another in a hospital emergency room you may have quite different ideas about what represents an 'appropriate' level of detail in questioning, or how quickly an interview needs to be completed for this to be 'reasonable'. Usually it is unrealistic for the teacher to try to prepare students to perform well under all possible circumstances. Careful thought is needed to decide just what a reasonable standard would be.

3. Notice how helpful specific examples are when you need to explain the reasons for your ratings to other teachers or to students. They can help you make your evaluations objective and understandable. However, such useful details may be quickly forgotten unless you make brief notes on them soon after they occur. An anecdotal record of the student's performance will be most useful if you include descriptions of actions that are representative of the student's usual performance, not just those that represent unusual triumphs or disasters. Exceptional incidents can give you convincing evidence of the student's learning, but they should not make you overlook the usual pattern of the student's actions if these reflect a quite different level of mastery.

4. Try to be consistent in the standards you use. Few things confuse and frustrate a student as much as being told at an early stage in her training that her performance of a particular task is excellent, only to be told later by the same teacher that the same performance is unacceptable. This can easily happen if you change your standards in mid-training. One source of this inconsistency is that teachers often use one or more of three very different types of standard:

- *Normative* standards that call for grading students 'on the curve' by judging how the individual student's performance compares with that of most other students at this point in their training

- *Individual* standards that compare the student with himself and focus on how much he has progressed since an earlier evaluation

- *Competency* standards that consider what quality of performance is needed for safe and effective independent action and tell us how close the student is to this practical goal.

Pity the poor student whose instructor shifts from one type of standard to another without explanation. The safest approach is to formulate a logical competency standard and then stick with it. This eliminates the 'moving target' presented by a standard based on the performance of others or on the student's level of experience. Competency standards tell you what you most need to know—whether the student's work is good enough for you to let him do the job independently. This focus need not prevent you from doing secondary evaluations as you think about whether a student is progressing towards acceptable competence as quickly as you expected, or whether his work deserves special recognition because it is clearly superior to that of most other people in a specified comparison group. However, the primary concern needs to be with achieving the competency goal and you will need to be clear both in your own thinking and your communication with others if your evaluation is based on a different standard.

5. Finally, try to make an exchange of views on standards and ratings a regular part of your future work.

- Case conferences, and clear documentation of teaching goals and accomplishments in the patient's record, can help you compare notes on standards and evaluations with other staff.

- Sharing your standards with students, asking them to assess their own performance, and taking time to compare ratings and discuss standards can be equally helpful.

- Grading conferences with other supervisors to review the standards you use and compare the ratings assigned students for whom you share responsibility can help you discover if your evaluations have become unrealistic or unfair.

Both thoughtful practice and critical feedback from colleagues are needed to maintain skill in evaluating the performances you observe.

USING EVALUATION TO COUNSEL STUDENTS

Accurate evaluation of student achievement is an essential part of good teaching, but to be productive these judgments must be communicated to the student and used as tools for planning and guiding future instruction. The first chapter of this Handbook includes one exercise concerned with the use of student evaluations to plan instructional activities (Exercise 2). Another exercise (Exercise 3) examines strategies the instructor can use for giving students reinforcement while they practice a new skill. Several references in the bibliography for this chapter suggest how evaluation forms can be designed to help a group of teachers coordinate their work with an individual student or to provide an administrative record to document achievement. All these are important methods for connecting evaluations with the rest of the teaching process. However, there is one other method for using evaluations to help students learn that is so frequently used and potentially valuable that it is singled out here for special attention. This is the evaluation conference or 'feedback session' in which student and instructor set aside a few minutes to talk about what the student has been doing, evaluate progress, and review strengths and weaknesses.

Such counseling may be scheduled in advance at regular intervals and review the students' work over a period of several days or weeks; or be less formal, occur spontaneously, and focus largely on an activity the student has just completed. Whatever their scope, these exchanges are most helpful if they are treated as opportunities for constructive planning in which instructor and student share their ideas about how things are going and what to do next. Their purpose is not simply for the supervisor to point out errors and announce future activities, it is to work with the student to analyze observations and explore alternatives.

As with most other teaching methods, the most effective way to use formative evaluation conferences depends a great deal on the setting, the student's level and preferences, and the types of skills he is trying to learn. However, the Guidelines summarized in the list attached to Exercise 22 provide a good basis for giving feedback in many situations. Exercise 22 will let you practice translating these general guidelines into practical action, and should help you evaluate some of your own present practices in counseling students in relation to a collaborative model of formative evaluation.

GIVING EFFECTIVE FEEDBACK

You will need to work with at least two other people to do this exercise.

Allow at least 40 minutes to finish all the tasks.

The exercise begins with evaluation of a simulated interview of a patient by a student. It then proceeds through a series of short conferences during which each member of your group will take a turn at trying to follow the attached *Guidelines for Giving Effective Feedback* as you counsel another group member on his performance.

The sequence of activities will be:

1. A simulated interview of a patient by a student—observed and evaluated by the student's clinical instructor

2. A feedback conference between student and instructor to discuss the student's performance during the interview

3. A feedback conference between the instructor and another staff member who observed the conference with the student to discuss how well the instructor followed the feedback guidelines

4. A feedback conference between the student and the staff member to discuss how well the staff member followed the feedback guidelines

5. General discussion by the group.

TASK A **Form a work group and assign roles**

Your group should have at least three members. If your group is larger than this the other members will not have a chance to practice giving individual feedback, but can try to apply the guidelines during the general discussion.

Decide who will take each of the following roles:

- student

- patient (this person can also play the part of the other staff member)

- clinical instructor.

TASK B **Plan the simulated performance**

Decide on the following elements of the role playing simulation:

- the patient's characteristics (e.g. diagnosis, age, sex, cooperativeness and any other personal qualities you think are important)

- the student's field of study or job description, level of experience and personal characteristics

- the purpose of the interview

- the setting in which it takes place.

The interview may consist of any series of questions a health professional might ask a patient for the purpose of planning the patient's care or monitoring his progress. Choose something with which all members of your group have had some recent experience. The questions should take at least 5 minutes to complete.

Assume that the instructor is present to observe but does not comment or participate while the interview is in progress.

TASK C **Review the rating criteria and feedback guidelines**

The student interview should be evaluated using the rating criteria and form attached to this exercise. If you have done Exercise 21 you will recognize them as the criteria you used then. If you have not seen the criteria before, take time to study them now.

During each of the feedback conferences the person who is giving feedback should attempt to follow the *Guidelines for Giving Effective Feedback* attached on a separate page. Review them before the role playing begins. They reflect a particular approach to counseling students with which you may not entirely agree. Keep track of any questions or reservations you have, but try to follow all the guidelines as fully as possible during your counseling session.

TASK D **Present and evaluate the simulated interview**

The role playing performance should last *at least 5 minutes.*

If the interview has not been completed *after 10 minutes, interrupt* it and assume this is as much of the student's performance the instructor has a chance to observe.

The instructor should use the following ratings to record his/her evaluations of the student's performance:

Excellent	— If this aspect of the student's interview was without error and included something that was unusually valuable and reflected a high level of skill
Acceptable	— if the interview met this criterion fully enough to make the questioning useful and acceptable to the patient, even if there were some minor errors or omissions
Unacceptable	— if the interviewer consistently failed to do this or if attempts to do it were so flawed it significantly interfered with the usefulness of the interview or was upsetting to the patient.
Uncertain	— if the observed performance provided too little opportunity for actions related to this criterion to assign it a rating.

Use the back of the rating form to make notes on any specific things the student did, or failed to do, that you felt were important in assigned ratings.

The student may be asked to use the interview criteria to assess her own performance if you wish.

TASK E **Present and evaluate a student–instructor feedback conference**

Allow a maximum of 10 minutes for this session.

The instructor should decide, and tell the group, where and when the conference is being held.

As the instructor talks with the student about her performance during the interview, the instructor should attempt to follow the *Guidelines for Giving Effective Feedback*. The group member who takes the part of another staff member (this can be the same person who earlier played the patient) should try to evaluate the instructor's success in following those guidelines.

TASK F Present and evaluate a feedback conference between the instructor and a staff observer

Allow a maximum of 10 minutes for this.

As these two people talk about how well the instructor followed the Guidelines, the group member who played the student should evaluate how well the staff observer follows the guidelines in her comments and questions to the instructor.

TASK G Present and evaluate a feedback conference between a staff observer and student

Allow a maximum of 10 minutes, and, as in the previous feedback sessions, see how well the student does when she gives the staff observer feedback on her compliance with the guidelines.

TASK H Discuss your observations and reactions with other group members

By the time you have gone through this cycle of three feedback conferences you may have both questions and opinions about the guidelines you were asked to follow. Take time now to discuss these. If some members of the group did not have a chance to take part in a mock conference, let them comment first on what they observed. Consider the following questions:

- Did you feel any of the guidelines were unclear, unrealistic or unnecessary?
- Did any seem especially helpful when you tried to give feedback?
- Were any especially helpful when you received feedback?
- Can you propose any other guidelines that should be added?
- Are these guidelines equally appropriate under all circumstances?
- When might you want to do something different? Why?

GUIDELINES FOR GIVING FORMATIVE EVALUATION

The feedback you give should be:

1. *Individualized.* Tell each student how he or she is doing rather than spending time discussing how 'most' students do, or even comparing this student's performance with that of another.

2. *Goal related.* Focus the discussion on the student's progress towards clearly specified performance objectives. Be sure the student understands what those objectives are and how his/her performance is being judged.

3. *Diagnostic.* Identify specific strengths and weaknesses rather than simply making global comments about overall performance. Anecdotal comments or examples often help to clarify. When problems arise in mastery of complex skills, work with the student to analyze his/her performance to figure out where the difficulty lies.

4. *Remedial.* Before the session ends try to work out with the student a practical plan for future activity that will help to maintain present strengths and remedy weaknesses.

5. *Collegial.* Collaborate with the student in reaching conclusions and planning future action; *listen*, be flexible, give the student time to put his/her thoughts into words, recognize that the student knows things about himself/herself you do not. Both your verbal and non-verbal behavior and the setting in which you meet with the student will have an important influence on your success.

6. *Positive.* Be sure to mention the things the student is doing right. You may also need to identify errors but be certain that's *not* the only thing you do. Try to arrange positive consequences of the student's actions to support your verbal feedback.

7. *Liberating.* Help the student learn to assess his/her own performance and to feel confident doing so. He/she will need to provide his/her own feedback when you are no longer available to do this.

8. *Selective.* Don't try to cover everything at once.

9. *Timely.* Try to give feedback as soon as possible after the student's practice performance. Give it after each attempt at first, but reduce the frequency of your feedback as the student progresses towards mastery and independence.

10. *Reciprocal.* Use these sessions to get ideas about your own strengths and weaknesses as an instructor. Remember that if a student is having problems you may need to make changes in what you are doing to help him/her improve.

OBSERVATIONAL RATING FORM

Skill evaluated: Carries out effective formal and informal interviews of clients to gain information needed for planning or evaluation of care.

Rating criteria	Rating
A. Makes a well-organized attempt to secure all pertinent information.	_____overall
• Asks questions on all important topics at an appropriate level of detail	_____
• Restates client response when necessary to clarify or summarize meaning	_____
• follows a logical progression without seeming inflexible	_____
• Completes the interview in a reasonable time.	_____
B. Uses effective verbal communication.	_____overall
• Expresses questions in simple and unambiguous sentences using terms the client understands	_____
• Avoids 'leading' questions and restatement of responses that 'put words in the client's mouth'	_____
• Speaks audibly and without irritating verbal mannerisms	_____
• Interprets the client's verbal responses accurately.	_____
C. Establishes and maintains good rapport with the client throughout the interview.	_____overall
• Begins the conversation by putting the client at ease	_____
• Uses body posture, eye contact and gestures that suggest attentiveness, approachability and acceptance	_____
• Acknowledges and shows acceptance of client responses	_____
• Allows the patient time to answer thoughtfully and to ask questions of his/her own.	_____

Notes

FEEDBACK ON EXERCISE 22

The feedback you received during this exercise should have helped you assess how able you are to use this particular approach to giving students feedback. However, the exercise is also intended to make you think in more general terms about techniques for formative evaluation. If you have not already discussed them in your group, think now about some of the issues this teaching method involves.

1. Both you and your students may need a good deal of practice before you feel comfortable using a collaborative model for feedback conferences. A more traditional approach in many educational programs is for these conferences to be directed by the teacher and focused primarily on pointing out shortcomings in the student's work. Making the collaborative approach work is not easy, even if you are enthusiastic about its potential advantages. Following these guidelines calls for a variety of complex communication and interaction skills. Among the most important is the ability to express empathy and to establish a climate in which both student and teacher feel it is safe to express doubts, admit error, enjoy success and disagree freely. Sometimes a few comments by the supervisor acknowledging that a task was difficult or confusing can do a lot to tell the student the teacher knows the job wasn't easy. Admission by the teacher that she too has made mistakes, and criticisms that are directed at the performance not at the student as a person, also may help. However such jobs as giving honest feedback to a student who is highly defensive—or to one who is unusually passive—require a wide array of interaction skills. This is an area in which most of us could benefit from continued study, practice and critical feedback.

2. Getting off to a good start is especially important. If you want the student to contribute freely, some of the time you will need to let her speak first. One way to do this is to begin the conference by encouraging the student to talk about her observations before you present your own. It is not enough to ask 'Can you think of anything else?' or 'Do you agree with that?' after you have completed a lengthy and authoritative analysis of her performance. On the other hand, completely non-directive questions, such as 'Well, where should we begin?' or 'How do you think you're doing?', may be intimidating to a student who is not used to this sort of exchange. The guidelines presented in this exercise are general, and each can be effectively carried out in many different ways. Deciding exactly what to do to get the conference started on a collaborative note is only one of the many points at which you will need to choose actions suited both to the student's level and to your own personal style.

3. Of course you may feel the collaborative approach outlined in the guidelines simply doesn't fit you and the setting in which you teach. This exercise will have been worthwhile even if you reject many of the guidelines so long as it provokes you to formulate some of your own and think about why you prefer them.

4. Even if you do believe a collaborative approach to feedback conferences has many advantages, you will need to use it selectively. Time pressures, interruptions and competing interests will raise many questions about when this type of formative evaluation is best. For example:

   - In this exercise the feedback you gave concerned just one performance of a specific professional task. You seldom have the luxury of being this focused in your real counseling ses-

sions. A variety of topics often demand attention, and the need to be selective and maintain some logical organization in discussion is essential. The use of written forms for recording evaluations can help. Especially if these forms describe the criteria by which learning will be judged, and are given to the student in advance, they can help you get your discussion started quickly, keep it on track, and remind you of points that should not be skipped even if you do take much of the conference to discuss other topics.

- Although the emphasis in this exercise has been on using supervisory conferences to give feedback, this is not the only thing that matters. Such meetings also provide some of your best opportunities for giving information and explanations. When the teacher is herself a highly skilled clinician, a problem or question raised by the student can open the door for a tutorial that is directly related to the student's immediate concerns. When such a 'teachable moment' occurs, don't waste it in the mistaken belief that didactic instruction is always out of place in a feedback session. This is one of the many points at which you must decide which has highest priority—giving feedback or information.

- Usually it takes only a few minutes to tell the student what you think of her performance and suggest what she should work on next. Engaging the student in mutual review and planning may take much longer. When time is short you probably will be tempted to use the few minutes you have making sure the student knows of any serious errors in her work, hoping her strengths will be obvious without your pointing them out. Many teachers use a fairly authoritative style in giving feedback early in the student's training, and plan to progress to a more collaborative style after she has mastered some of the basics. Unfortunately, if you do this you may find that you have run out of time before this change is made, or that once the student has gotten used to your authoritative style requests for self-assessment seem intimidating.

To use supervisory conferences effectively you will need to maintain a sensible balance between asking and telling, praising and criticizing, leading and listening. This will be easiest to do if you take time *before* the conference begins to set priorities for the different things you might try to accomplish. If you have seen some serious flaws in the student's work, and know your meeting must be short, you may want to control the conversation yourself and ignore peripheral topics, however interesting they may be. On the other hand, if you feel this is a time when helping the student learn to evaluate his own work is of special importance, deciding that before the meeting begins may make it easier for you to bite your tongue and hold back on your own comments to give the student a chance to practice taking the initiative.

FOSTERING SELF-ASSESSMENT

The first three exercises in this chapter describe things you can do to improve the accuracy and usefulness of your evaluations; but this is only the first step. The teacher's job is to help students get off to a good start. However, much of our students' most valuable learning takes place long after we have lost direct contact with them. The case was forcefully described by Kelly West when he wrote:

In medical education the practical utility of instruction is limited by several considerations, including the following:

1. Only a small portion of the current body of medical knowledge can be taught in four years.
2. Much of the knowledge which will be employed in the student's future career is not known today and, therefore, cannot be taught.
3. Not all that is taught is learned.
4. A small part of what is taught is erroneous.
5. A small portion of what is taught will soon be obsolete.
6. The physicians of the future (including family physicians) will be specialists. Thus, some of what they learn will have limited relevance to their careers.
7. Of that which is taught, and learned, and relevant, much is quickly forgotten.

It is evident that to an ever-increasing extent the quality of medical care will be determined by the physician's capacity to acquire new knowledge and acumen, while attempts to teach the medical student all he will need to know will become increasingly futile.[3]

While West's comments were directed at medical education, his concerns seem equally relevant for teachers in most other health professions. The capacity to acquire and use new knowledge has been given a variety of elaborate names. Some call it the capacity for independent growth and self-renewal, others prefer to speak of the potential for life-long learning. Whatever label you use, this clearly is an area of skill with which you must be concerned. The patients, staff and students we teach have almost reached the point when they must function on their own. We can do few things as valuable as trying to make sure they are prepared to continue learning after the day of their discharge or graduation arrives.

This task is not easy. Developing independent learning skills requires just as much instruction,

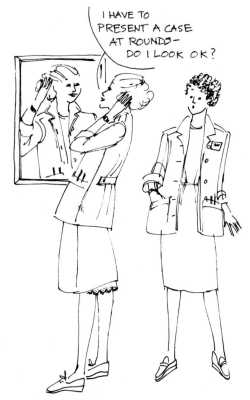

I HAVE TO PRESENT A CASE AT ROUNDS — DO I LOOK OK?

practice and nurturing as any of the other complex things we teach. This means we must set aside a significant amount of time to make sure the student is prepared to do for himself all those things his teachers have done in the past:

- decide what he needs to learn

- arrange activities and locate resources that will help him learn

- judge his own progress and provide his own feedback.

Doing all this calls for an impressive array of special skills and attitudes. For example, Hesburgh et al[4] mention the following things they feel colleges and universities must teach their students in order to prepare them for life-long learning:

- intellectual curiosity

- independence and self-direction

- confidence in their own ability to learn independently

- a base of knowledge and skills flexible enough to permit students to move into related or complementary fields and to adapt to change in their own field after graduation

- ability to use largely unstructured, unprogrammed educational opportunities.

The clinical setting provides a wealth of opportunities for helping patients, staff and fieldwork students acquire these skills and values. Some of these have been mentioned in other sections of this Handbook. For example, some of the things you can do to prepare the people you teach to become independent learners are:

1. Establish a relationship with your students that shares power and responsibility and shows in large ways and small that the student is regarded as a reasonable person whose ideas and preferences matter. (In this Handbook Exercise 13 on Sharing power and 19 on Role models and relationships provide examples of how this can be done.)

2. Give students choices in the instructional activities you arrange; and, as their preparation progresses, ask them to take the initiative in suggesting and designing activities for themselves. (Exercise 12 on Contracting, and Exercise 24 on Preparing a list of learning options, provide guidelines and practice for several techniques that can help you do this.)

3. Find out what your students already have learned through their earlier studies and life experience and validate this by:

- commenting on its value

- adapting the instruction you plan to build on what each student already knows. (Exercises 4 and 8 in Chapter 2 emphasize the need to do this by talking with students about their past experience, interests and concerns before deciding what we will try to teach them.)

4. Arrange some experiences that give your students a chance to 'muddle through' ambiguous problems or unclear situations. Let them both solve problems for themselves, and pick out and define problems they think need to be solved. Give them the freedom to improvise, experiment, explore and discover. (The feedback section for Exercise 16 includes a brief comparison of teacher-structured and student-structured experiences and some

comments on the Discovery method of instruction.)

5. Take time for conversations with your students that go beyond simple reporting of their activities and encourage them to:

- examine the way they went about making important decisions

- explain why they did or did not do specific things and why they think one method for solving a problem worked when another did not

- integrate what they are learning now with things they have been taught earlier.

(This sort of teaching relies more on questioning than on 'telling'. The feedback section for Exercise 18 includes some suggestions for types of questions you may find useful.)

6. Arrange for your students to take part in activities centered around discussion with their peers. Encourage them to practice getting and giving information and feedback by talking with others who share the same responsibilities or problems. For patients and their families self-help and support groups often serve this purpose admirably. When they are not available the clinical teacher often can schedule several patients with similar problems at the same time and provide a setting in which they can compare notes about solutions to the problems they share. For professional staff and fieldwork students the opportunities for such peer teaching are even more numerous, and often can be built into necessary patient care activities to save time and make them a customary part of day-to-day work. Some familiar examples of such discussions are:

- giving reports at the time of shift changes on a nursing unit or reviewing cases with a colleague who will take over your case load while you are on vacation

- planning and carrying out quality assurance programs such as an outcomes audit

- case conferences and rounds, particularly if these encourage free discussion and critical review of alternative approaches to intervention or varying interpretation of signs and symptoms

- group research projects
- periodic staff journal club sessions.

This is only a small sample of the ways we can teach our students to teach themselves. Some of these methods are particularly useful for helping students learn to take initiative, others for building skills in solving unfamiliar problems independently. However, we must recognize that all these efforts ultimately depend for their success on another essential skill not specifically mentioned so far—skill in self-assessment. It provides both motivation and direction for independent learning. Without honest and accurate self-assessment our 'graduates' may become careless or out of date without realizing it, and may waste valuable energy in efforts to learn that are irrelevant to their real needs. Self-assessment is a necessary piece of nearly every step in independent learning:

- To be self-starting the graduate must be willing and able to critique his own skills and recognize if they are becoming rusty or obsolete.

- To be self-directed the graduate must be able to identify his own interests, judge his own capacities for growth, and evaluate what available learning opportunities have to offer.

- To be self-paced the graduate must be able to assess his own rate of progress realistically.

- To be self-steering the graduate must be able to diagnose specific strengths and weaknesses in his own performance and provide his own guiding reinforcement.

Unfortunately, self-assessment is a topic on which the research literature in education is curiously silent. Many authors, notably those with a special interest in adult education, have written with passion about the importance of allowing adult learners to chart their own educational course, and a variety of studies have attempted to identify personal and professional characteristics associated with health workers' participation in formal programs of continuing education. However, little basic research has been undertaken so far to determine how adult learners actually go about assessing their own educational needs, and which methods are most fruitful. Descriptions of methods for teaching self-assessment skills are equally skimpy. The most widely reported efforts to encourage self-assessment involve development of self-assessment tests by professional organizations, and efforts by individual clinical instructors to have students use teacher-prepared rating forms to evaluate their own work. These do engage the student in some important aspects of evaluation, but they do little to encourage the student to decide for himself which of his skills need evaluation and by what standards his performance should be judged.

The topic of self-assessment is ripe for serious study. Until we learn more about it, however, we can only assume the student must go through the same series of steps as the teacher when he attempts to evaluate his own learning. One way to analyze this process is to try a self-assessment of your own. Exercise 23 will let you do just that by reviewing some of your own current evaluation practices.

EVALUATING STUDENT ACHIEVEMENT: A SELF-ASSESSMENT INVENTORY

This exercise can be done entirely on your own. However, if you wish, you can complete the first five tasks independently and then discuss your reactions with a group of other clinical teachers. Allow at least 25 minutes for Tasks A through E and another 20 minutes for discussion.

TASK A **Complete the attached self-assessment inventory**

This inventory lists 10 teacher activities often recommended as needed for fair and useful evaluation of students. Think about what you have done during the last 6 months during your evaluations of the patients, staff and fieldwork students you teach. Then use the scoring key on the inventory to rate the frequency with which you do each of the things listed.

TASK B **Review any activities you do only occasionally**

Think about what determines when you do this and when you don't.

- Does it depend on how much time you have? Is this something you agree is useful but not of such high priority that you feel you have to do it even if you're rushed?

- Does it depend on the student? Is this something you do only with 'difficult' students? Is it something you do only near the beginning or the end of your work with most students? Are there some types of students who respond well to this and others who do not?

- Does it depend on the type of content you are teaching, or the setting in which this occurs?

TASK C **Review any activities you seldom or never do**

Try to decide why this is so. Is it because you:

- think this is inappropriate and prefer a different approach

- teach in a situation that makes it impractical or unnecessary?

- don't know how?

- simply never thought about doing it?

TASK D **Describe any other evaluation activities you think are important**

The list in the inventory may seem incomplete. Think about other things you believe are necessary for sound evaluation of student achievement.

EXERCISE 23

TASK E **Think of some specific observations that support your beliefs**

Select one of the actions you do frequently and feel is important for good evaluations, and one you seldom or never do and feel is not worthwhile. What evidence from your own experience supports these opinions? Try to recall specific occasions on which you tried each of these actions. What happened, and what makes you feel this represents the type of result you usually can expect from this action?

TASK F **Discuss your ratings and reactions with other teachers if you wish**

Talking about this exercise with several other clinical teachers is a good way to clarify your own thinking and get different points of view on a controversial topic.

- If the members of your groups teach in different settings or teach different types of students, see whether this determines the way you carry out evaluations.

- Explain your rationale for doing some things only occasionally or never to see whether your logic makes sense to others.

- Talk about how you think the inventory should be revised.

Then turn to the feedback section for some general comments.

EVALUATING STUDENT ACHIEVEMENT

A Self-Assessment Inventory
How often do you do each of the 10 things listed below when you evaluate your students?

Use the following ratings to describe your present practice.

Usually or always .... score 10
Occasionally .... score 5
Seldom or never .... score 0

Your score   Evaluation activity

_____ 1. Base evaluations on observation of how the students perform important tasks rather than on impressions of such general traits as their attentiveness, initiative or problem-solving ability.

_____ 2. Judge the student's performance by comparing it with a pre-determined standard that describes the essential characteristics of an acceptably safe and effective performance.

_____ 3. Explain to students early in instruction how their work will be evaluated and what standard you expect they will achieve.

_____ 4. Actively encourage students to suggest how they would like to be judged and to evaluate their own performance.

_____ 5. Monitor the students' progress at frequent intervals to decide whether they will reach an acceptable level within practical time limits for teaching.

_____ 6. Confer with at least one colleague each time you adopt a new standard or complete a major evaluation of an individual student to see whether your goals and judgments are realistic.

_____ 7. Keep a record on each student that includes notes describing specific incidents you feel reflect significant strengths or weaknesses in his/her learning.

_____ 8. Talk with each student at frequent intervals to review progress and problems and plan future instructional activities based on this evaluation.

_____ 9. Document a summary of your evaluations and the standards on which they were based so other teachers can read and interpret them without difficulty.

_____ 10. Review the results of your student evaluations to look for areas in which your own teaching methods may need to be changed.

EXERCISE 23

FEEDBACK ON EXERCISE 23

The self-assessment you did for this exercise was fairly simple and quite incomplete. Comprehensive self-assessment requires the same series of basic steps as those listed at the start of this chapter for the teacher. This exercise lets you practice some of those steps, but not others. For example:

- The Inventory provided a *focus* for your self-assessment by asking you to start by reviewing your current practice in 10 specific areas. Left to your own devices, you might have taken quite a different approach. Some of the 10 recommended actions may have seemed unclear, others impractical or irrelevant for someone in your situation. The list probably overlooked at least one other action you think is important. One reason to be suspicious of rigid rules for performing complex tasks is that different situations often call for very different procedures. However, a list of recommendations such as this can help you get started on a useful self-evaluation. Taking a self-assessment test published in a professional journal, hearing an expert present her ideas on how a particular job should be done, asking a co-worker what he thinks is important, can remind you of points you should not overlook and provoke you into defining a focus of your own. If this Inventory stimulated you to think about how you want to evaluate your own assessment of students it served a useful purpose no matter how strongly you may have disagreed with some of the recommended practices.

- Measurement of your actual practice relied on your recollection of the frequency with which you perform different actions. Your perception of your own behavior may have been biased or uncertain. Particularly if you are an experienced teacher, you probably do many important things intuitively. This can make it difficult to visualize and classify your actions. You may have felt quite uncertain about some ratings because the description of the activities on the inventory was confusing. Or you may try to do some of these things frequently, but have doubts about how successful you are. Keeping a simple log or tally of your evaluation activities over a period of several weeks, or reflecting in detail on what you did with two or three different students, can help you check your general impressions. Asking co-workers or the students themselves to tell you what they believe you do can help too. Whatever source of data you use to describe your actual performance, try not to be vague. Ask yourself and others for specific examples of your actions rather than basing your ratings on a general, unanalytical impression.

- The most significant missing piece in this self-assessment exercise was the lack of any explicit *standard* to help you judge your actual performance. Even if your perception of what you usually do is accurate and specific, how are you to decide what this means? The rating key asked you to record how frequently you do each of the 10 recommended activities, but frequency may not be the most important determinant of effectiveness. You may have asked such questions as:

  — Is the ideal score on each activity 10—or would it really be better to do some of these things only occasionally?

  — What is a 'passing' score? At what point should I recognize that my overall performance is seriously flawed and needs improvement?

  — What do I want to consider beside how often I do these things? How could I measure the *quality* of my evaluations?

FEEDBACK

To be fully independent in your self-assessments you will need to select a focus, set standards, measure your own performance, and judge your achievement for yourself. As you do this perhaps your best source of guidance is your everyday real work. Inventories and suggestions from colleagues can help you generate ideas, but eventually these will need to be tested against reality in your own particular situation. Ask your students which of the things you do in your evaluations they find helpful and which they do not. Ask yourself what difference you expect your evaluation procedure to make and then turn back to reality to see whether you actually get the results you expect . . . and, of course, as you do all this keep track of self-assessment methods that seem to work well for you so you can try to pass these important skills on to your students.

NOTES TO CHAPTER 5

1. Bloom B S, Hastings S T, Madaus A F 1971 Handbook of formative and summative evaluation of student learning. McGraw-Hill, New York
2. Delbeque A, Van de Van A 1976 A group process model for problem identification and program planning. In: Benis W, Benne K, Chin R, Corey K (eds) The planning of change, 3rd edn. Holt, Rinehart and Winston, New York, pp 283–295
3. West K 1966 The case against teaching. Journal of Medical Education 41: 770
4. Hesburgh T, Miller P, Wharton C 1973 Patterns for lifelong learning. Jossey-Bass, San Francisco

6 RESPONDING TO INDIVIDUAL DIFFERENCES

Students are not all alike; effective teaching must respond to individual differences. This maxim has been repeated over and over in the earlier sections of this Handbook. Clearly, teachers are not all alike either. Just as students differ in their starting level, interests, learning style, abilities and plans for the future, teachers vary widely in their talent, experience, personal traits, teaching philosophy, and in the resources and constraints of the settings in which they work. Identifying these individual differences is important; but it is only a first step. We must build on this analysis to plan a practical approach to teaching that capitalizes on individual strengths and compensates for individual weaknesses.

DIFFERENCES AMONG STUDENTS

Let's look first at how this might be done from the student's point of view. Individualized learning demands flexibility in instructional activities that lets them be matched to at least some of the personal needs, interests and abilities of each student. Four very different dimensions of instruction must be considered:

● *Purpose*

Even a highly varied group of students usually shares some common learning needs, but around this core of uniform goals we often need to provide substantial choice. Differences in present interests, future plans and practical resources may make some objectives essential for one student and irrelevant for another. A selection of *optional objectives* is one important ingredient of an individualized learning program.

● *Process*

Some students learn best alone, others profit greatly from studying in groups; some progress most easily if they begin with a theoretical framework, others find theory mysterious until they have practical grounding in specifics. These and many other differences in individual learning style make it logical to offer students *learning activity alternatives* that permit them to match at least some features of the instructional process to their own preferred pattern.

● *Pacing*

Differences in the speed with which students master new knowledge and skills is a particularly obvious source of diversity. If all students are required to progress through assigned activities at the rate we believe is 'average', some are sure to be frustrated because they could progress faster, while other will do poorly or fail, not because they are incapable of mastery, but simply because they need a little more time. *Elastic time requirements* for the duration and frequency of practice of key skills can let us adjust for these differences and allow each student some opportunity to move at her own speed.

● *Placement*

Placement of each student through assignment of activities appropriate for his individual starting level requires a practical system of *competency assessment*. Such individual evaluation also enables students to bypass instructional activities they don't need, and lets us monitor individual progress towards achievement of a predetermined standard of acceptable performance.

Attempting to do all this may seem logical—but unrealistic. Clinical teachers do try to adjust instruction when individual students have problems or when a student is clearly gifted and able to take on unusual responsibilities. However, these adaptations often are made intuitively. The precious moments available for deliberate planning of instruction are most likely to be invested in designing experiences many students can use. Efforts to individualize instruction are limited, not because we feel this is unimportant but simply because it seems to 'take too much time'. This is, of course, a problem clinical teachers share with their counterparts in the classroom. Small wonder that in recent years a wide variety of methods has been developed to diversify instruction without making the process unworkable for the instructor. Most of these methods require some initial investment of time to develop flexible instructional materials. Usually, however, this time can be recovered when the materials are put to use because they allow students to get some of the information, practice and feedback they need independently, without the instructor being present. Projects and independent studies, learning contracts, computer assisted instruction and self-instructional booklets or audiovisual programs, pairing of students with complementary skills for peer teaching or shared work on assignments, and learning resource centers that offer students a choice of media for receiving information, are only a few of the methods that enjoy current popularity in many academic programs. Most have promise for individualizing clinical instruction as well; but, in fact, few are widely used in this setting. The obstacles are obvious. Many clinical teachers are employed primarily to give patient care and have difficulty freeing blocks of time for initial development of elaborate self-instructional materials. Few clinicians have the specialized facilities or advanced skills in in-structional design some of these methods require. However, there are some simple things most clinical teachers can do to expand on their intuitive responses to individual student differences. One practical way to begin is to select a type of learning that is important for many of the students you teach and then prepare brief written descriptions of several different ways the individual student might choose to work on this objective. This sort of à la carte menu of instructional activities does little more than present the student with the sort of information about available choices many teachers customarily share during conversations and conferences. However, putting the choices in writing has several advantages. It:

- encourages the teacher to consider options that otherwise might be overlooked
- frees the teacher from time-consuming repetition of basic information about available choices
- allows students more time to think about the method they prefer
- provides a skeleton to which more extensive self-instructional materials can be added in the future if time permits.

When the objectives and instructional activity options are appropriate for students in more than one specific setting, these simple written lists have an additional advantage. They can be exchanged with other clinical teachers and so serve to increase the variety of options students can be offered while limiting the work any one teacher needs to do to explain these choices. The following sample shows one way in which such a list of options can be presented.

Exercise 24 outlines a series of steps you can follow to develop a summary of learning activity alternatives of your own.

_____ *Sample* _____

LEARNING HOW SALT AFFECTS YOUR BLOOD PRESSURE

Your doctor has recommended you limit the amount of sale (sodium) in your diet as part of a total program to control your blood pressure. To help you learn how to do this you have an appointment to meet with a dietitian from our Hypertension Clinic staff on

_____ (date)   at _____(time)

She will go over your usual diet and talk about any changes that may be needed.

Before you have that meeting we would like to be sure you understand how salt affects blood pressure and why limiting the amount of salt in the food and drink you consume is important.

Here is a list of several different things you can do to learn this. Please read the list and then let the Hypertension Clinic secretary know which one of them looks best to you. Choose the one you prefer and the secretary will arrange for you to get any materials or appointments you need.

To learn how salt affects your blood pressure and why it is important to limit the amount of salt in the food and drink you consume you can do *any one* of the following:

1. Read a short booklet about *Salt and Your Blood Pressure* published by The Heart Association. The booklet is 6 pages long. It is free and you may keep your copy. The clinic secretary will give you the booklet. Let her know whether you would prefer one written in English or in Spanish.

2. Watch a 10 minute television program on 'Salt in your diet—why is it important?' The program was made by the staff of our Hypertension Clinic. It is shown every day at 10:00 a.m. and again at 2:30 p.m. in the hospital's Health Education Center located near the pharmacy. The program is free and friends or members of your family may watch it with you if you like. The clinic secretary can give you directions for getting to the Education Center. You do not need an appointment for this.

3. Attend a 45 minute class along with several other patients who also need to limit the salt in their diet because of high blood pressure. This class is scheduled from 3:00 to 3:45 p.m. every Thursday and is taught by the dietitian from the Hypertension Clinic. After she explains how salt affects your blood pressure, the dietitian will tell you about several kinds of food that contain a lot of salt and should be avoided. She also will show you how you can find out how much sodium (salt) there is in canned and packaged foods at your market. You will have a chance to ask any questions you have about these subjects and to talk with other patients. We make a $5 charge for attending this class. One family member or friend may come with you at no extra charge. You will need an appointment to go to the class. The Clinic secretary will make the appointment for you.

4. *Or*—you can take a short Test-Yourself quiz to find out whether you need to learn more about salt and your blood pressure. You may already have learned everything you need to know about this from a family member or friend, in a class at school, or by reading or watching television. If you think you already know something about this subject, ask the Clinic secretary for a copy of 10 short questions we think you need to be able to answer. It will take you only a few minutes. The secretary also will give you a page showing the correct answers. When you finish answering the questions you can score your-

self. You do *not* need to tell your score to anyone else. The purpose of this quiz is simply to help you decide whether you need to do one of the first three things on this list. There is no charge for the quiz, and you may keep the questions and the answer page.

PREPARING A LIST OF LEARNING OPTIONS

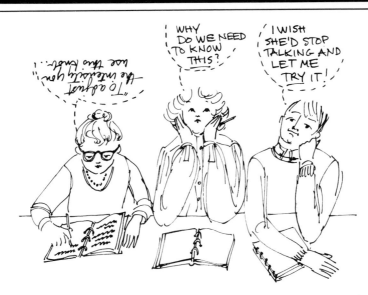

You can do this exercise alone, or work on it with a partner or small group of other clinical teachers. Allow at least 40 minutes to complete all the tasks. If you are working with a group, you may want to allow longer so you will have time to hear everyone's ideas.

Your job in this exercise is to prepare a written list describing several alternative activities your students could carry out to work on one important instructional objective. The end result should be a page or two of information you could give these students to tell them what options are available.

TASK A Decide what type of students will use this list

The sample shown earlier in this Handbook was prepared for use by adult out-patients in the Hypertension Clinic of a general hospital who have recently been told by their physician they should limit their sodium intake. You may prefer to design a list of learning options for staff trainees or fieldwork students. Whatever your preference, you will need to decide:

- what category of students your teaching involves, and
- where and when you assume you are working with them.

Try to choose a type of student with whom you have worked often enough to have a good idea of some of his individual differences. If you are doing the exercise with a partner or group, choose a type of student and a setting for instruction with which you all have had recent contact.

TASK B Select a learning goal for the list

Review the objectives you usually have for this group of students. Select one that you feel is especially important and that:

- involves tasks performed frequently in this setting so that opportunities for practice are plentiful

- is broad enough so it might be worked on in any of several different ways
- is easy to describe in terms these students will find easy to understand.

TASK C Make a preliminary list of possible learning activities

Begin by thinking about different things you have arranged for students to do in the past that have seemed to help them achieve your objective. Then go on to see if you can think of other activities that seem practical to arrange and useful for acquiring this type of learning. Jot down a few words about each activity as you think of it.

If you are working with a partner or a group, begin by making a list of ideas of your own and then compare your lists to see if others have thought of worthwhile activities you overlooked. You may want to compile your ideas into a single master list if you all work with similar students in very similar settings.

Your purpose here is simply to think of many different ways in which a student could work on the objective you chose. Don't worry about detail at this stage.

TASK D Edit your list to emphasize significant choices

Now re-work your original list to narrow it down to a selected list of alternatives that offers students choices in areas where their individual needs and preferences are most likely to vary. There is no 'magic number' for the variety of choices you should offer, but for practice in this exercise you should try to describe *at least three* significantly different options.

These activities don't all have to be exclusively concerned with the one objective you've chosen as the focus of your planning. You may want to suggest some activities that allow the student to work on several other types of learning at the same time. The important thing is to be sure each activity on your edited list gives the student a good chance to do things directly related to your objective, and that these activities are different from each other in ways that let each student choose a method of learning matched to some of her personal needs, interests and abilities.

Some examples of the types of choices you may want to build into the options on your list are:

- when to do the activity
- how often to repeat it
- how much support or supervision to have
- whether to work alone or with one or more fellow students
- whether to be told how to carry out the activity or be asked to figure out how for herself
- whether to be an active participant or a spectator
- whether to work primarily with abstract ideas or concrete things and events
- whether to be asked to consciously analyze experiences and observations or to respond to them intuitively as a whole
- whether to concentrate on learning one thing at a time or to work on this objective at the same time as several others
- how much authority to take during interactions with other people
- from what source to get any information she needs (e.g. reading, asking others, etc.)
- how frequently and from what source to get feedback on her performance.

Try to include the types of choices your past experience with this type of student has shown you are important, but don't overlook choices you may simply never have thought about before.

Regardless of the number and types of choices you provide, be sure to do one other thing:

- Include in your list of options some method the student can use to find out whether she needs *any* further work on this objective if she thinks she may already have reached an acceptable level of mastery.

TASK E **Describe the options in terms the students understand**

As you edited your initial list of ideas you should have decided which specific characteristics of each activity are of special importance. Now it is time to put a summary of your plan into writing so you can give it to students when the time comes for them to work on this objective. The sample presented earlier in this Handbook suggests one way of doing this. Use a different style and format if you wish but try to write your descriptions at about the same level of detail as those in the sample. The students may need additional instructions in order to carry out the activity they choose. Don't try to cover everything in this list. Simply describe the options in enough detail so important differences among the alternatives are easy to see and students will know enough about what each activity involves to make a realistic choice.

Avoid complicated sentences and technical terms the students may not understand.

Remember to include practical information about such things as how long the different options will take, when scheduled events will occur, and how to arrange to do the activity they select.

TASK F **Write a brief introduction**

To complete your list, write a short paragraph describing the overall purpose of these activities and explaining who the list is for. This is also a good place to explain that the student only needs to do *one* of the activities on the list and may choose whichever he prefers.

As with the activity description, write this in simple terms as if you were talking with one of the students in person.

Write the introduction in at the top of the list.

If you are working with a partner or group, and have decided to pool your ideas in a single list that combines everyone's ideas, make certain each of you has a copy of the end result. You will need this to get feedback.

FEEDBACK ON EXERCISE 24

If you are currently teaching the type of students for whom this list of options is intended, the best way to get feedback is to pilot-test it with several of your own students. Give each student a copy of your list when you reach the point at which it seems logical for her to work on the objective with which it is concerned. Add to your written explanations only if the student asks for more information or appears confused. Then go ahead and arrange for the activity the student chooses.

The following list of guiding questions will help you evaluate both the merits of the activities you selected and the clarity with which you explained them.

A. As you work with the student to arrange or supervise the activity she chose, try to talk with her about:

1. The *clarity and completeness of your descriptions*. For example, ask:

   - Do the written descriptions tell you enough about the different activities for you to tell which one you like best?

   - Are any of the descriptions confusing?

   - Is there anything else you'd like to know about any of the activities before you decide which you want to try?

2. The *significance of the differences in the activities* you planned.

   - How do you feel about being asked to choose an activity?

   - Does it matter to you which of the activities you try, or do they really all seem about the same?

B. After the student has completed the activity she selected, try to talk with her to find out what she thinks about:

1. The *accuracy of your written description* of that activity.

   - Did this activity turn out to be what you expected?

   - Did the written description you were given describe it fairly?

2. *How will the activity* the student selected *fit her individual needs*.

   - How did the activity go for you?

   - Did you feel as if doing this really helped you learn what the written list said you would?

   - Were there any things you especially liked about the activity you chose?

   - Were there any things you wish could have been different?

   - Overall, how well did this activity match the way you personally feel you learn best?

C. After you have tried using the list with at least five or six different students, think back on their reactions and ask yourself:

1. *How much variety was there in the choices* students made?

   - Did they all choose the same thing?

   - Was one of the activities you thought good turned down by everyone?

2. *Can you explain why they made the choices they did?*

   - Were the activities few students chose much more demanding or less familiar than the others?

   - Did the activities many students chose have some obviously attractive feature?

   - Were you surprised by the preferences of individual students? Could you have predicted what they would choose from the way they have responded to other parts of their training with you, or on the basis of their personal characteristics and background?

The questions suggested here are simply examples of ways you can explore how students reacted to your list of options. They will seem more natural if you select the points that fit your situation best, and if you express the questions in your own words.

If you are not currently teaching this type of student—or—if you would like preliminary feedback on your list before using it with students, you can use the same list of questions as the framework for a critical review by another clinical teacher. To do this:

- Explain to your colleague that you are trying to give students choices about the way they go about learning so they can match their instructional activities to their own personal needs and preferences,
  and
  that you hope this written list will give them the information they need to choose an activity without your taking time to give each of them the information in person.

- Make sure your colleague knows:
  — what type of student you intend the list for
  — in what sort of setting it will be used
  — what objective the activities are designed to achieve.

- Then ask the colleague to try to imagine he is a student, and to think about which activity he would prefer.

- When he has made a choice, go through the questions under A and B from the student pilot testing suggestions, and ask your colleague if he has suggestions on how the options or descriptions could be improved.

The main purpose of this exercise is to encourage you to offer your students alternatives and to help you identify some of the types of individual differences you may need to consider in doing this. Putting the options in writing certainly isn't essential. However, if you find this works well for you, think about expanding on the list you composed here. Some clinical teachers have developed files or notebooks that contain a number of these 'menus' for selecting a personal learning program. Others have designed more extensive self-instructional materials to which students can turn when they wish. Program and materials to help students evaluate their own level of mastery, interests and preferred learning style are also in use in some clinical teaching units. To do these things you will need skills that go considerably beyond those called for by this exercise. The bibliography suggests some references that can help you learn more. Meanwhile, remember, even a few simple choices described in a simple written list can help you get started on the important business of responding to individual student differences.

DIFFERENCES AMONG TEACHERS

Now let's look briefly at the other side of the coin. If we shift our attention from differences in how students learn to differences in how teachers teach several things are obvious.

- The first is that variations in teaching style are necessary and desirable. There is no one best way to teach—no style that is superior in all situations.
- Secondly, we must take several quite different factors into account in deciding what teaching style to use at any given moment. Differences among students are important, but they are only one of the things we must consider. Selection of an effective approach also depends on
  - the type of subject matter being taught
  - the constraints and resources of the specific teaching situation and
  - the technical expertise, personal skills and philosophical beliefs of the individual teacher.

Many features of the average teacher's personal style are probably the result of conscious or unconscious imitation. We may teach the way we were taught simply because no other approach ever occurs to us. Or, we may selectively adopt techniques we have seen used effectively by 'master teachers' whose reputation and results we admire. This first-hand knowledge of different styles can be usefully expanded by reading books and attending classes that endorse and explain a particular approach to teaching. Adult education methods, the inquiry approach, teaching for mastery, the problem-solving curriculum, values- clarification exercises, programmed instruction, discovery learning and behavior modification . . . these and a wide variety of other special techniques all represent potentially useful tools. Our problem is not to decide which one is best, it is to develop some logical system for selecting, combining and adapting such tools to fit our own talents, our students' needs, and the demands of a specific subject and teaching situation. A first step towards developing such a framework for flexibility is to look at some of the many choices of style you make each time you teach a student, and then to review your actions to analyze what factors seem to guide your decisions. Exercise 25 will give you a chance to practice doing this.

ANALYZING YOUR OWN TEACHING STYLE

In this exercise you will be asked to use a series of 15 short rating scales to evaluate the way you teach. Each scale represents a continuum between two quite different approaches to teaching. Your job will be to mark the point on each scale that reflects the emphasis you believe you place on each approach.

It will only take you a few minutes to mark the 15 scales. However, the exercise suggests several different options for marking and interpreting them. Depending on the options you choose, completing the exercise may take as little as half an hour *or* be something you work on now and then over a period of many months.

Some options can be done alone, others require participation of several students.

TASK A **Familiarize yourself with the rating scales**

The scales are attached to this exercise. Read them over to see what they include and how they are arranged. Although the scales do refer to many different dimensions of teaching style, they certainly do not cover all the ways in which teaching may vary. You may think of additional choices you feel are equally important. If so, *add scales* to represent these in the space allowed for this at the end of each group of five scales.

The two different approaches at the ends of each scale are not mutually exclusive. In other words, you do not have to do all one and none of the other. If you feel you give *both* approaches *equal* priority, put your mark in the center of the scale. If you feel you choose one *most* of the time but occasionally do the other, put the mark closest to the approach you use (or would like to use) most often.

You may want to make several copies of the scales to use for the different rating activities.

TASK B **Decide on a frame of reference for your ratings**

Because your teaching style may change depending on the type of students you are instructing and the setting in which you do this, your ratings will be easiest to interpret if you think about the way you teach in a specific situation.

• Choose a type of student and teaching situation with which you have had considerable recent experience.
• Be specific enough so you can visualize yourself at work and think of specific examples of your teaching related to the different approaches described in the scales.

TASK C **Rate your present teaching style in this situation**

Think about what you *usually* do when you teach the type of student you have selected in the setting you designated . . . not what you wish you did, what you *actually do at the present time*.

Mark the point on each scale that best represents your approach. Do this by writing a capital letter *A* above the scale line at the point you choose.

No matter which options you choose in Task D, do this rating of your *actual* style first.

TASK D **Complete one or more of the following additional ratings**

Each of the options listed here is intended to stimulate your thinking about teaching style by comparing the ratings of your present style with ratings carried out from a different point of view.

Do as many of the options as you wish. They are listed in the sequence in which it will probably be easiest to complete them if you do more than one.

Regardless of which optional ratings you do, please remember *there is no one right way to teach.* Neither you nor any students or fellow teachers with whom you compare ratings should feel that these represent an evaluation of how good a teacher you are. The purpose of this task is to help you think not just about *what* you do when you teach but *why*.

- Take time to 'talk to yourself' and to anyone else who works on the exercise with you to share your ideas about why you assigned the ratings as you did.
- Try to think of specific examples of real actions that reflect your approach. This can help you clarify for yourself and others how you have decided to interpret the very general terms used to describe contrasting approaches on the style scales.

Additional rating options

1. Continue to focus on the type of student and setting you used in Task C, but this time mark the scales to show the way you feel you would perform if you were free to be an *ideal* teacher. Mark these sections with the symbol *I*.

    Earlier comments emphasized that there is no one ideal style. That's true; but for a specific setting and type of student you should be able to suggest what approach you think is usually most promising. If you find your ratings for an ideal style are different from those for your actual present approach, try to explain why this is so.

2. Rate your actual teaching again, but this time shift your focus to a *different type of student and setting.* Mark the scales with the symbol *D* to show the approach you believe you actually take when you teach the alternate situation.

3. Ask one or more of your *students* to complete the scales to record their perception of your approach to teaching. Obviously, you should select students who fall in the group you defined in Task B. Ask them to record their ratings with the symbol *S/A*.

4. Ask one or more of your *students* to mark the scales to record their views of what the *ideal* teacher would do. If you also ask the same students to rate your actual approach you may need to reassure them that it's OK if there are some differences between the two sets of ratings.

    Ask the students to mark these ratings with the symbol *S/I*.

5. Ask several *other clinical teachers* who work with the type of student you selected in Task B and who teach in that same setting to rate their own *actual* style. Compare them with your own and with each other. These ratings should be marked with the symbol *O*.

6. Or—identify the ratings you have collected with today's date, and file them in a safe place. In a year or two take a clean copy of the 15 scales and *repeat* your earlier ratings. Then get out the original versions and see what has happened to your actual teaching style and to your ideas about teaching.

WHAT KIND OF TEACHER?
A Teaching Style Inventory

Role and relationships

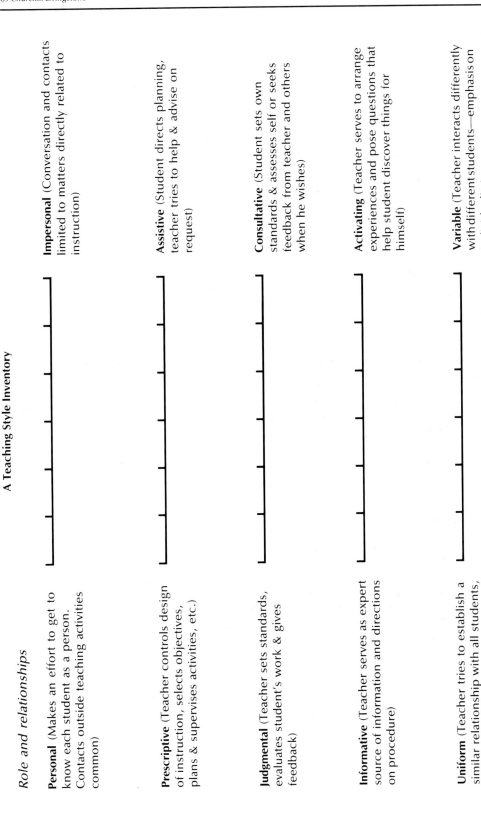

Personal (Makes an effort to get to know each student as a person. Contacts outside teaching activities common) — **Impersonal** (Conversation and contacts limited to matters directly related to instruction)

Prescriptive (Teacher controls design of instruction, selects objectives, plans & supervises activities, etc.) — **Assistive** (Student directs planning, teacher tries to help & advise on request)

Judgmental (Teacher sets standards, evaluates student's work & gives feedback) — **Consultative** (Student sets own standards & assesses self or seeks feedback from teacher and others when he wishes)

Informative (Teacher serves as expert source of information and directions on procedure) — **Activating** (Teacher serves to arrange experiences and pose questions that help student discover things for himself)

Uniform (Teacher tries to establish a similar relationship with all students, emphasizes impartiality) — **Variable** (Teacher interacts differently with different students—emphasis on individuality)

EXERCISE 25

Nature of content emphasized

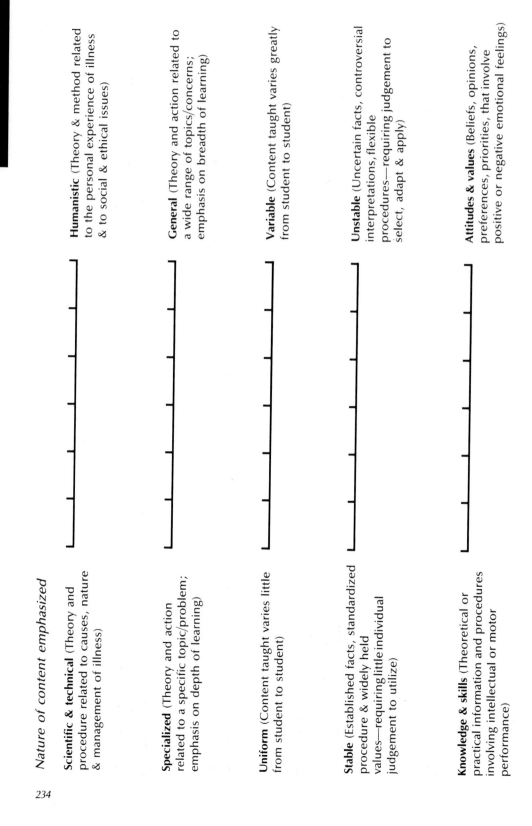

Humanistic (Theory & method related to the personal experience of illness & to social & ethical issues)

General (Theory and action related to a wide range of topics/concerns; emphasis on breadth of learning)

Variable (Content taught varies greatly from student to student)

Unstable (Uncertain facts, controversial interpretations, flexible procedures—requiring judgement to select, adapt & apply)

Attitudes & values (Beliefs, opinions, preferences, priorities, that involve positive or negative emotional feelings)

Scientific & technical (Theory and procedure related to causes, nature & management of illness)

Specialized (Theory and action related to a specific topic/problem; emphasis on depth of learning)

Uniform (Content taught varies little from student to student)

Stable (Established facts, standardized procedure & widely held values—requiring little individual judgement to utilize)

Knowledge & skills (Theoretical or practical information and procedures involving intellectual or motor performance)

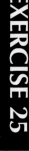
EXERCISE 25

Practical (Ability to perform useful procedures effectively, safely and effectively—emphasis on knowing how)

Futuristic (Ability to adapt to and help create future change)

Intuitive (Ability to see things as a whole, deal with complex and subtle aspects of a situation instinctively)

Divergent (Ability to raise questions and generate a variety of ideas)

Instrumental (Mastery of knowledge, skills and attitudes that are useful for achieving practical goals)

Type of learning emphasized

Theoretical (Ability to explain, interpret, formulate and apply general principles & hypotheses—emphasis on knowing why)

Current (Ability to do the things they need to do today)

Analytical (Ability to reason logically, break a problem apart, and explain rationale for actions—conscious and deliberate thinking)

Convergent (Ability to select the best answer or solution to a problem)

Personal (Development as an individual, personal enjoyment, growth & self-knowledge)

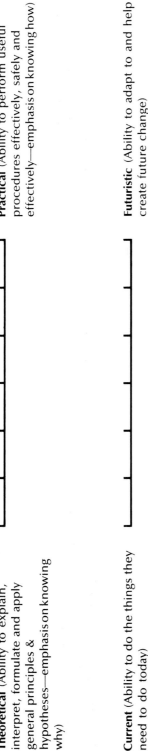
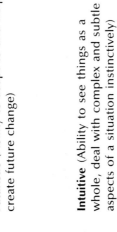
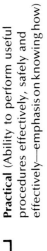
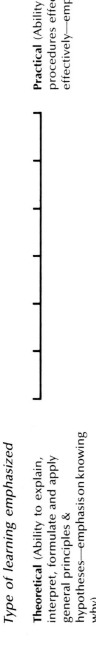
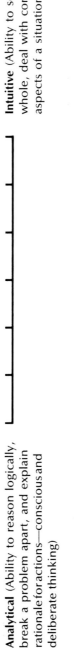
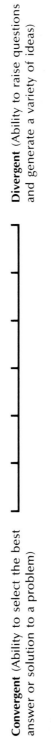
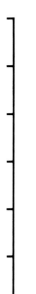
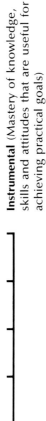

EXERCISE 25

FEEDBACK ON EXERCISE 25

Your best source of feedback on this exercise will be the thinking you do on your own and the conversations you have with other teachers and students. Your own interests and reactions should determine the direction of these discussions. However, here are some broad questions you may want to consider.

1. How accurate are your perceptions of the way you actually teach?
    If you tried option 3, comparison of your own actual style ratings with those of your students should provide some useful reality testing.

    If you found it difficult to think of concrete examples of things you do that reflect the style you believe you use—you may be fooling yourself. For example, if you rated yourself as placing a great deal of emphasis on teaching attitudes and values, you should be able to think of some specific things you actually do to accomplish this.
2. Do you have a logical rationale for the style you prefer?
    If your reasons are vague and your preferences strong, this is probably worth further thought. Intuitive preferences can be very sound, but as a student of the art and science of teaching, you should be able to do better than, 'I've just always done it that way'. 'That's how I was taught', or 'I don't know. .it just seems to work'.
3. Can you explain the source of any differences you found between your ideal and actual style ratings?
    If you found such differences, try to decide whether this is the result of:
    — external obstacles: lack of time, restrictive policies, limited resources or other situational constraints.
    — internal obstacles: lack of ability or training needed to do what you think is ideal, or perhaps simply lack of motivation or confidence to try something different.
    Some obstacles may be possible to overcome, others may be insurmountable. However, the first step towards achieving your own ideal style is a realistic analysis of any problems.
4. How much do you appear to adapt your style to meet the needs of individual students and different situations?
    — If you tried option 3, was there some variety in the way individual students felt you had worked with them?
    — If you tried option 2, did the approach you preferred seem to change as the type of students and setting changed?
    — If you tried option 4, did individual students disagree with one another about the style they rated as ideal?

This exercise provides only a very superficial look at a fascinating and important subject. In the references mentioned in the bibliography you will find other, very different models for describing and analyzing teaching style and for matching style to individual differences in learning. This is a subject you should continue to explore for many years to come.

FEEDBACK

7 PUTTING THE PIECES TOGETHER

Most of this Handbook is concerned with the planning and presentation of individual lessons—with the design of a single lecture, the supervision of one practice session, the evaluation of one performance. Specific learning experiences are the building blocks of our instruction, and much depends on the skill with which each lesson is crafted. However, effective teaching requires more than good individual lessons. We also need a master plan, an overall organizational framework that helps us put the pieces together so they add up to the pattern of learning we seek. Most clinical instruction involves a series of lessons, some extending over only a day or two, others covering a period of many weeks. To organize these into a cohesive whole we must plan not just lessons but a curriculum or program.

The principles of curriculum design are far too complex to explore thoroughly in this Handbook, but they are much too important to ignore completely. This chapter is intended, therefore, to draw your attention to this topic, give you a very general idea of its scope, and stimulate your interest in learning much more about this side of teaching.

DIMENSIONS OF ORGANIZATION

Organizing separate learning experiences into a logical program or curriculum raises three distinct categories of questions:

- Some concern the *sequence*[1] in which different topics or skills should be introduced. For example, you may need to decide:
  — Where should I begin? What should I save for last?
  — In what order should I have the student work on the different skills she needs to master?

  — What is the best time to have students try to learn this?
- Others concern *continuity* and the opportunity for repeated practice of skills that cannot be mastered in a single attempt:
  — How much time should I allow for students to learn this?
  — How many other chances is the student likely to have to work on this?
  — How quickly can I plan to progress to more demanding assignments?
- And a different group of questions concern *integration* and grouping of the different experiences to form a cohesive whole:
  — How can I help students see how the different things they are asked to learn are connected?
  — What sort of relationships should I emphasize?
  — Which skills should the student learn concurrently, and which need to be learned one at a time?
  — Should I include this topic in what I teach, or would it be more logical as part of what someone else teaches these students?

To answer such questions we must review the various objectives and experiences with which our day-to-day teaching is concerned, and try to find a logical pattern of organization that considers two dimensions. To answer questions about cumulative learning and progressions we need to focus on important differences among experiences and objectives: differences that could provide a logical basis for deciding on sequence and continuity. This is often referred to as the vertical dimension of organization for it tells us how we might progress from beginning to advanced skills or from initial attempts to full mastery within a single area of learning. When our questions concern integration or grouping of learning experiences, however, our attention must turn to the horizontal dimension as we look for similarities, for common elements that can serve to tie separate experiences together and help us avoid wasteful fragmentation.

These are rather abstract concepts. To see how they work when you try to apply them, do Exercise 26. It asks you to try to organize a sample of small objects rather than a group of different learning activities, but the organizational process is much the same for both tasks.

DESIGNING AN ORGANIZATIONAL SYSTEM

You can do this exercise alone, but it will more interesting if you arrange to do it along with several other people with whom you can compare results. These other people do not have to be clinical teachers or health professionals.

You should be able to finish your individual work on the exercise in about 10 minutes. Allow another 15 or 20 minutes if you want to compare work with other people (Task D).

TASK A Look briefly at the attached picture

Attached to this exercise is a drawing of 15 small objects. These are the things you will be asked to organize. Assume they all come from various desk drawers at a nursing station or office in which you sometimes work.

Look at the picture for a moment to see what it includes, but do *not* discuss the objects or their organization with anyone else.

TASK B Decide how these objects could be divided into groups

These are the rules you should follow in doing this:
1. You must have at least two groups.
2. Every group must include at least two objects.
3. All 15 objects must be assigned to a group—no 'leftovers'.
4. Each group should be based on some characteristics all the objects assigned to it have in common and you should be able to state what this shared quality is.
5. You may *not* have a 'miscellaneous' category.

If you are doing the exercise alone you may find it easiest to take a pair of scissors and cut a copy of the picture into pieces so you can move them around to try out different groupings.

However, if you are doing this along with other people *do not* move the object pictures, or point to them, or talk about them as you work. Work silently. The whole purpose of doing this with others is to compare the different approaches you use when you do this task independently.

TASK C Now, decide how these objects could be lined up in a logical order

Here your job is to think of a systematic basis on which these 15 objects could be organized in a row stretching across the table.

You should have a single line that includes all 15 objects, and be able to explain the logic behind your progression by saying: 'I've put the things in sequence from––to––.'

As in Task B, if you are doing the exercise with others, work silently and independently as you figure out your organizational principle.

TASK D **Compare the way you organized the objects with the methods others used**

If you have been working alone, the feedback section will give you ideas on several possible systems for grouping and sequencing these objects.

If you are working with others, ask one person to tell you how many groups she had, and to list the objects in each group *without* explaining what she thinks the objects in each group have in common. See if you can figure out the logic for these groupings. Then let her do the same with your groups. If you have cut the picture into pieces you can describe your system simply by moving the pieces into groups without saying anything.

Use the same method for showing each other the sequence in which you lined up the objects. See if you can figure out what principle each person used.

The purpose of this exchange is simply to let you see several different ways these objects could be organized, and to let you practice summarizing your organizational logic in words.

When you have finished, turn to the feedback section for some comments on how this organizational exercise is related to the work you must do to organize the instructional activities you arrange for your students.

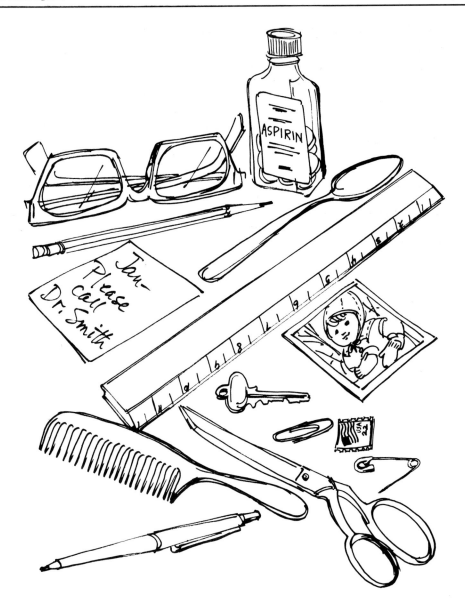

FEEDBACK

FEEDBACK ON EXERCISE 26

Organizing specifics into logical groups

Perhaps the most obvious thing about Task A is that it can be done in many different ways. You might have chosen any of a wide variety of shared qualities as the basis for grouping these objects. For example:

- You might have based your groups on some physical characteristic such as size, weight, predominant color, or whether the object has square corners, rounded corners or a mixture of the two
- Or you could have grouped the objects in terms of the type of material from which they appear to be made (metal, paper, mostly wood, etc.)
- The objects could be grouped by probable ownership (e.g. institutional property or personal belonging of a staff member)
- Or on the basis of their probable use.

These are only a few possibilities. Thinking of potential groupings is easy for both objects and learning activities. The difficult part of this organizational task is to find categories that will include *all* the components we need to put into groups, and to select the basis for grouping that is most useful.

In curriculum planning deciding what to do with 'left-overs' can be difficult. We often have some instructional objectives or experiences that we feel are important which don't seem to fit neatly into a group with the other things that concern us. Too often we end up with a lecture, fieldwork assignment or practice session that includes a hodge podge of all the odds and ends we haven't covered somewhere else. For students, these experiences are likely to seem pointless and confusing. Even if they involve several obviously important things, the lack of organization often impedes learning, dilutes motivation, and makes learning difficult to retain. Taking time to try to group material in a more comprehensive way can be very worthwhile. This can be done in any of several ways. For example, suppose you began trying to group the objects in this exercise on the basis of their most frequent use. You might have tried using three categories and made the following initial assignments:

Use=	Communication	Personal needs	Holding things together
Objects:	pencil	aspirin	paper clip
	pen	spoon	safety pin ,
	stamp	comb	
	phone message	eyeglasses	

Fine so far, but what should you do with the baby picture,
                              ruler,
                              key, and
                              scissors?
You could deal with these 'left-overs' by:

1. *Broadening the definition* of one or more of the original categories to add related qualities that allow you to include otherwise unclassifiable items. For example, you might expand the

'Holding things together' group to include things used to connect *or* disconnect different objects. This would let you assign the key and scissors to that group.

2. *Emphasizing some less obvious attribute* of some of the unclassified items to focus on qualities that make them fit an existing group. For example, you might assume the baby picture is a photograph of some staff member's son or child of a former patient. By thinking of this in terms of its value for meeting personal needs for affiliation you might feel you could combine it logically with the comb, spoon, aspirin and glasses. You might see the ruler as a device for recording size in commonly recognized units, and therefore a tool for communication. Expanding categories in this way can easily become far fetched, but even a contrived logic for organizing things can be better than complete lack of a pattern.

3. Looking for some quality the left-over items have in common and using this to *develop a new group* may help.

If you find several important instructional objectives or experiences simply don't seem to fit into any of the groups you have thought of first, the best approach may be to start from scratch and look for an entirely different logic for grouping. In clinical teaching we frequently add new things to the information and skills we have taught in the past. Sometimes these combine easily with the old material, but over time our 'curriculum' for patients, staff and students often becomes both overstuffed and fragmented. When this occurs, it can be very worthwhile to try to step back from our customary pattern of organization to try to think of new groupings that make it easier to pull old and new content together and help us avoid the repetition and confusion that so often goes with illogically organized teaching.

Selecting the system of grouping that is most useful can be equally challenging. The most important thing to remember is that our purpose in grouping is to make learning easier for the student. Too often our organization is determined primarily by such things as custom ('I've always taught that') or perceptions of expertise ('nurses are the ones who know most about that, they should teach it') when a different pattern might make much more sense to the student. For example,

- In deciding who will teach what to newly diagnosed diabetic patients we might consider having one person teach both how to alter sugar intake through careful selection of foods *and* how exercise can be used to influence consumption of sugar in the body. The patient will need to combine these in maintaining an appropriate balance. Even if traditionally these have been taught separately by a dietician and physical therapist, combined teaching might be more useful to the patient.

- If we want a fieldwork student to learn how to determine when patients or family are unable to 'hear' and accept unwelcome information about their condition, we might consider assigning the student activities that will let him work briefly with several such patients in a single day even though our customary pattern is to have the student carry broader responsibilities for only one patient at a time.

Functional categories for grouping activities can be especially useful. This means organizing instruction along the lines of the uses students will make of the information and skills we present. To do this requires a sensible analysis of the individual student's probable future activities. No single pattern of organization is likely to fit them all. Consider, for instance, the way books on human anatomy are organized. In some, the chapters or major sections are organized around different systems or types of tissue: cardiovascular system, nervous system, muscles, etc. In others, the organizational groupings are regional: upper extremity, back, head and neck, etc. The student of surgery is likely to find the regional atlas most useful as he tries to visualize the structures he will encounter as he makes a particular incision. The nurse trying to correlate clinical signs with pathophysiology in patients suffering from a specific digestive disorder may find the system-based grouping of information best.

Deciding on the basis for sequence also confronts us with a wide array of choices. In Task C, for example, you might have arranged the objects in order of their increasing weight, relative economic value, probable frequency of use, overall length . . . or any of a number of other dimensions. To plan a logical sequence we must look for some significant quality all the specific objects or activities have in common, but also one they possess to varying degrees. As in establishing logical groups, as you review the various different progressions you might use you need to:

- choose one that seems directly related to the student's needs and the way they will use the different things you plan to teach
- define it clearly enough so it is easy to tell where specific items should be placed on the continuum.

Vague descriptions of the progression are of little practical value. For example, fieldwork supervisors often describe the difference between the responsibilities they assign a beginning student and those they assign when the student is nearly ready to graduate by saying, 'Well, at first I only give them simple cases and easy things to do. Towards the end I expect them to cope with difficult tasks and really complex cases.' What does this mean? The problem is that it might mean many different things. One person might think of a task as 'easy' because it requires no special social or motor skills to perform; another might say easy tasks are those that are highly standardized and involve little or no judgement; a third might think of easy tasks as those in which speed of performance is not essential and modest errors are not critical. Your selection of easy and difficult assignments might be quite different depending on which of these many possible definitions you used.

In this exercise you were asked to think of a single set of groups, and only one principle for progression. In planning how to organize instructional activities you probably will want to use several different patterns in combination. For example, if you have already worked your way through many of the earlier chapters in this Handbook, you may have noticed it is organized in the following way:

- The guidelines and exercises are grouped into chapters based on different steps in the instructional process—the different tasks most clinical teachers frequently need to carry out. This grouping was selected because it focuses on responsibilities most clinical teachers have in common, regardless of their professional field or whether they primarily teach patients, staff or fieldwork students. Had the emphasis in the book been on *what* to teach rather than *how* to teach a different set of categories would have been more useful. . .perhaps one based on diagnostic groups (e.g. what to include in your instruction of patients with chronic lung disease). Or, chapters organized around different types of learning might be helpful (e.g. 'How to teach attitudes and values' or 'How to teach discharge planning'). Each pattern has its special advantages. Selecting one to use isn't always easy.
- The sequencing of material in the Handbook makes use of several different progressions. One is temporal. The various teaching tasks are presented in the order in which they usually need to be done (e.g. deciding what to teach before deciding what instructional method to use). The other principles for progression are more complex and include:
  — sequencing of the scope of concepts discussed from an early reductionist focus on specific, observable student behaviors to a later emphasis on more holistic, less tangible aspects of learning, such as learning styles
  — progression in the flexibility of techniques described from early emphasis on rather detailed description of step-by-step procedures for doing such things as writing objectives and carrying out task analyses to later presentation of more general guidelines for things such as giving effective feedback in which there are many different ways in which the general recommendations can be interpreted and applied
  — a shift in the source of feedback from early reliance on presentation of 'correct answers' by the Handbook to greater use in later exercises of guiding questions you can use to assess your own work or to get feedback from colleagues.

246

Although these were intended as the overall pattern for the book, at many points this logic is ignored because of expectations about how the Handbook will be used. It seems likely that many readers will use the book not by starting with the first chapter and working their way methodically through the exercises in the order in which they appear, but by sampling here and there to work with the particular exercises that fit their own interests. For this reason, the exercises were designed so each of them could be used entirely on its own. Some cross-referencing to other sections of the book is provided to suggest connections with related ideas. This sort of flexibility requires a considerable sacrifice in continuity and integration, but is necessary to reduce confusion if the expectation that many readers will sample rather than consume the entire book proves correct. In your own teaching you may need to make similar compromises—planning the sequence of instruction you prefer to build on previous learning you hope your students already will have, yet preparing yourself to change your plans if a student arrives with unexpected gaps in her skills.

Finally, the organizational pattern for the Handbook includes a component you were not asked to consider in Exercise 24. This is an overall framework or set of unifying concepts that attempt to pull the many pieces together into a cohesive whole. In deciding what to include in each chapter, as in deciding what to have a student do on any particular week of field work assignment, we must look for a constellation of differences and similarities that let us group specific activities logically. In designing an overall curriculum framework we must look for common elements in all these groups that we can use to emphasize how they are related. These elements may take the form of central questions, problems, concepts or beliefs. In clinical teaching we are particularly likely to use the individual patient and his problems as a unifying focus. For the student in professional fields such as occupational therapy or dietetics, whose early didactic instruction includes a bewildering array of courses in everything from sociology to biochemistry, it is in early work with individual patients that the pieces all begin to come together. As we supervise the student's efforts to assess the patient's problem and design a plan of care, we can help her draw upon the diverse knowledge and skills she has acquired in the classroom and laboratory. Recognizing the power patient problems have for helping students integrate learning, professional educators have developed various systems for bringing them into the curriculum at an early stage. Early clinical observation, simulated case problems, arrangements for each student to have a continuing, long-term contact with an individual patient or family all represent tools for accomplishing this. Perhaps the most fully developed system for using patient problems as the focal point for organizing instruction is the Problem Based Learning approach developed by Barrows and Tamblyn.[2]

Patient problems are only one of the integrating elements we can use. This Handbook, for example, has attempted to use several recurrent ideas as unifying themes. The most obvious of these is the view of the basic teaching—learning process discussed in Chapter 1 and summarized graphically in Figure 1. Specific teaching tasks, such as motivating students and providing feedback, are discussed, not just as discrete processes, but as interdependent components of a larger whole. Equally important is repeated emphasis on a series of broad maxims or beliefs about what teaching is and how it should be done.

- Teaching is more than simply organized presentation of useful information.
- Relevant practice and guiding feedback are essential for learning.
- Teachers seldom have enough time to teach everything that might be useful—selectivity is important.
- Flexibility is important, too. There are usually several good ways to do a good job.
- Students need to become independent, the teacher should help them learn the skills this will require.

Repetition of these themes in connection with each of the various aspects of clinical teaching allows them both to be emphasized and to be used to point out qualities the different teaching tasks have in common. As you read this explanation of the organizational logic for the Handbook

FEEDBACK

you may feel it didn't work as it was intended so far as you are concerned, that another pattern might have been more useful, or that some devices have been overused. As you invent your own systems for organizing your clinical teaching, you can profit from drawing on the ideas that textbooks and research in education can provide. However, you also need to test your design by talking with your students. Their feedback will be your best index of whether your groupings, sequences and integrating ideas are actually accomplishing what you hoped.

NOTES TO CHAPTER 7

1. The terms sequence, continuity, and integration are used here as they were defined by Ralph Tyler in his brief but immensely influential discussion of curriculum organization in Basic Principles of Curriculum and Instruction 1950 University of Chicago Press, Chicago
2. Barrows H, Tamblyn R 1980 Problem based learning: an approach to medial education. Springer Series on Medical Education, Vol 1. Springer, New York

ANNOTATED BIBLIOGRAPHY

CHAPTER 1 Teaching & learning process

To learn more about the learning process and how it can be applied in your day-to-day clinical teaching you may want to use several rather different categories of references.

A good place to begin is with one of the books on clinical teaching that includes a section on practical applications of learning theory. These references usually do not discuss alternative theories in great detail, but do provide a useful overview of main points. The practical guidelines derived from theory are useful and should help you see why analysis of learning process is important and which elements of the process might be most valuable for you to study further. Several particularly helpful references in this category are:

REDMAN B K 1988 The process of patient education, 6th edn. Mosby, Saint Louis
A fine overview of learning theory terminology and concepts combined with detailed examples translating various theories into specific techniques for teaching patients and families. Methods described range from operant conditioning to guided imagery, and applications are as diverse as teaching a child to swallow a pill and helping adults cope with anxiety prior to surgery. An extensive bibliography is provided.

O'CONNOR A B 1986 Nursing staff development and continuing education. Little Brown, Boston
A brief but informative description of three very different views of what learning is and how it occurs: stimulus–response associationism, Gestalt psychology and cognitive-field psychology. Implications of these theories for teaching are illustrated with useful examples from nursing staff education.

ALEXANDER M 1983 Learning to nurse: integrating theory and practice. Churchill Livingstone, Edinburgh
A succinct and informative overview of theory and research on the learning process. Guidelines for application are fairly limited, but the range of views discussed is wide.

ROSE G 1986 Approaches to learning. In: Hinchcliff S M (ed) Teaching clinical nursing, 2nd edn. Churchill Livingstone, Edinburgh
Combines general comparison of associative and cognitive views of learning, and a summary of internal and external conditions that influence learning process, with analysis of the part these factors play in clinical teaching to achieve such outcomes as psychomotor skills, problem solving and concept-rule learning.

As you continue your study of learning theory you may want to consult a text that provides a more detailed analysis of the psychology of learning and reviews some of the research on which various theories are based. Although the following references all give greatest attention to classroom instruction, they will help you identify some of the still unanswered questions about learning and suggest ways in which existing theory can be applied in higher education and in teaching adults.

HILGARD E, BOWER G 1975 Theories of learning. 4th edn. Prentice Hall, Englewood Cliffs, New Jersey
One of the most widely respected references on learning, this important text summarizes a wide variety of theory and related research. A chapter on theory of instruction suggests how principles inherent in theories can be applied by the teacher.

ENTWISTLE N, HOUNSELL D (eds) 1975 How students learn. University of Lancaster Institute for Research and Development in Higher Education, Lancaster

An important collection of readings on learning selected for their relevance for higher education, including papers by authors such as Brunner, Skinner, Gagné, Rogers and Ausubel. Some take a very intellectual view of learning, others emphasize the humanistic aspects of the process. Most include comment on practical implications for teaching.

BEARD R 1976 Teaching and learning in higher education, 3rd edn. Penguin, Harmondsworth
Includes an unusually broad chapter on the psychology of learning that provides a useful summary of the major differences between the views of Gestalt-field psychologists and those of the stimulus–response associationists.

GAGNÉ R 1977 The conditions of learning. Holt, Rinehart & Winston, New York
Describes conditions that affect human learning and relates these to the design of instruction concerned with five different types of learning: intellectual skills, cognitive strategies, verbal information acquisition, motor skills and attitudes. Comments on problem solving as a method of learning are of particular interest.

KLEIN S B 1987 Learning: principles and application. McGraw-Hill, New York
A detailed and easy-to-read review of major learning theories and the psychological research through which they have been developed and tested.

Finally, in addition to reading more about the various components of the processes of learning and teaching, take time to look at some of the more philosophical writings on this topic. Each presents an integrated way of thinking about these activities, an overall approach that usually is grounded in science but also depends heavily on common sense, experience and a general point of view on what teaching and learning are all about. These models differ widely from one another, but each can help you consider possible systematic connections among the diverse factors studied by learning psychologists. The references listed here are only a small sample. For additional suggestions see also the bibliography for Chapter 6.

KADUSHIN A 1976 Supervision in social work. Columbia University, New York
Includes a superb chapter on educational supervision built around six general maxims concerning conditions that promote learning. These broad principles are stated in

common-sense terms and emphasize such points as the need to present new content within a framework that has meaning for the learner, and the value of considering each student's uniqueness as a learner. Each maxim is accompanied by a series of clear, logical suggestions for its application. The ideas presented seem equally applicable to work with students or with staff trainees.

REILLY D, OERMANN M 1985 The clinical field: its use in nursing education. Appleton-Century-Crofts, Norwalk, Connecticut
Presents an elegant conceptual framework for thinking about learning and teaching that is particularly applicable to education of professionals in a clinical setting. This holistic model incorporates such varied topics as the role of concept formation, experiential learning and problem solving, and the influence of cognitive style. Separate chapters provide detailed discussion of the nature of cognitive, affective and psychomotor learning, and suggest practical applications of this theory during clinical instruction.

ROGERS C 1969 Freedom to learn. Charles Merrill, Columbus, Ohio
A classic reference that presents many of the ideas that are the foundation for much current writing on adult education. The author's 'theory of learning' is presented as a series of personal assumptions about the process of learning rather than as conclusions based on formal research. Suggestions of methods teachers can use to facilitate learning are based on these assumptions. In addition to its importance in the literature on non-authoritarian teaching, this reference provides a remarkable example of teaching methods logically derived from a holistic view of learning.

CHAPTER 2 Defining the purpose of teaching

Defining the purpose of your clinical teaching calls for two quite different processes: first you must decide what you want to accomplish, then you must explain this in terms other people can understand. For an overview of both tasks, begin with one of the following:

ROSE G 1986 Aims and objectives. In: Hinchcliff S M (ed) Teaching clinical nursing, 2nd edn. Churchill Livingstone, Edinburgh
Explains the difference between general statements of purpose and objectives that specify exactly what will be expected of students, and

provides helpful guidelines for both writing and using objectives.

BECKS S J, LEGRYS V A 1988 Clinical laboratory education. Appleton and Lange, Norwalk, Connecticut
Includes summaries of the taxonomies of objectives by Bloom, Krathwohl and Simpson (see later section of this bibliography) along with practical suggestions on how to write objectives and sensible comments on how they can be used.

CAPUT D Z 1976 Instructional objectives. In: Ford C, Morgan M (eds) Teaching in the health professions. Mosby, St Louis
Includes brief but practical explanations of several methods for establishing educational needs, a summary of the uses and components of behavioral objectives, and descriptions of several systems for classifying learning. Of particular value are the many examples applying these ideas to objectives for students in a variety of health professions.

To learn more about techniques for analyzing your students' learning needs and interests see:

O'CONNOR A B 1986 Nursing staff development and continuing education. Little Brown, Boston
Provides information on a wide variety of methods for assessing staff learning needs. These range from surveys and checklists to job analysis, performance appraisal and records audit. Helpful comments on responding to future trends in practice and on interpreting the results of assessment are of special value.

RANKIN S H, DUFFY K L 1983 Patient education: issues, principles and guidelines. Lippincott, Philadelphia
Provides an exceptional variety of ideas on how to establish instructional goals for patients. The emphasis throughout is on cooperation rather than compliance, and the model of goal setting presented is one that depends on sensitive exploration of individual patient and family concerns and resources, and uses a process of mutual involvement of patient and practitioner in setting objectives. Among the features that make this book especially valuable are the beautifully outlined guidelines for assessing the needs of the patient and for evaluating the resources and practices of the institution in which instruction is provided. Also of special interest are the many case examples that illustrate how general recommendations and theory can be converted into practical actions.

NARROW B 1979 Patient teaching in nursing practice: a patient and family centered approach. Wiley, New York
Outlines a comprehensive yet practical approach to goal setting for patients that draws on such sources as textbooks, patient interviews and evaluations of individual learning styles and readiness to learn. Of extra interest are the logical comments on assessment of the strengths and limitations of the teacher and teaching situation, two factors seldom addressed in the literature on selection of objectives.

DEA K L, GRIST M, MYLI R 1982 Learning tasks for practice competence. In: Sheafor B, Jenkins L (eds) Quality field instruction in social work. Longman, New York
Clear, detailed examples illustrate selection of objectives for clinical fieldwork through identification of tasks for which students will be responsible as graduate professionals and analysis of the knowledge and skills each task requires for competent performance. Attention is given to both current and expected future demands in the field using a process that can be readily applied in most professional disciplines.

MAGER R, BEACH K 1967 Developing vocational instruction. Fearon, Belmont, California
Describes a series of practical steps for setting training goals that begins with job analysis, and then moves through analysis of component tasks to identification of required knowledge and skills. Both the frequency with which tasks must be performed and the difficulty of mastering each step are considered. Examples of analyses are drawn primarily from the skilled trades (e.g. electronic repairman), but the process is equally applicable to many health fields. This is an interesting complement to the reference by Dea et al in which most tasks discussed are highly varied and complex.

As you turn from thinking about what students need to learn to analysis of what you have to offer, a discussion of the special characteristics of the clinical teaching environment may help you be realistic in identifying important assets and constraints. Several references that provide this are:

REILLY D, OERMANN M 1985 The clinical field: its use in nursing education. Appleton-Century-Crofts, Norwalk, Connecticut
Includes a valuable chapter on the clinical milieu as a learning environment.

BALLANTYNE E F 1986 Ward learning: opportunities and problems. In: Hinchcliff S M (ed) Teaching clinical nursing, 2nd edn. Churchill Livingstone, Edinburgh
> Uses examples based on nursing education in a British hospital but the ideas discussed have very broad application.

INFANTE M S 1975 The clinical laboratory in nursing education, 2nd edn. John Wiley, New York
> Identifies 14 essential elements that should be embodied in the design of student experiences in the clinic and discusses how each can be used, or misused. Comments point out the strengths of the clinical environment for fostering such skills as critical thinking, problem solving and inquiry; but also emphasize things the teacher must do to take advantage of these resources.

WIEMER R B 1984 Student transition from academic to fieldwork settings. In: Commission on Education of the American Occupational Therapy Association, Guide to Fieldwork Education. American Occupational Therapy Association, Rockville, Maryland
> A short but thought-provoking discussion of both tangible and intangible differences between the classroom and practice environments and of the pressures these can create for students.

As you begin to translate the results of these assessments into specific statements of instructional intent you will need to analyze exactly what types and levels of performance students need to master by the time you complete your teaching. Several references that will help you think of verbs that focus clearly on the actions you hope to see are:

MAGER R 1972 Goal analysis. Fearon, Belmont, California
> A good natured, down-to-earth workbook that urges you to avoid 'fuzzy', abstract terms describing very global purposes, and shows you how to focus instead on clear description of the specific actions you want students to be able to perform.

BLOOM B S (ed) 1956 Taxonomy of educational objectives: the classification of educational goals. Handbook I: the cognitive domain. David McKay, New York

KRATHWOHL D R, BLOOM B S, MASIA B B (eds) 1969 Taxonomy of educational objectives: the classification of educational goals. Handbook II: the affective domain. David McKay, New York

SIMPSON E J 1972 The classification of educational objectives in the psychomotor domain. In: Contributions of behavioral science to instructional technology: the psychomotor domain. Gryphon Press, Mt Ranier, Maryland

These three references describe widely used systems for classifying different types of learning and for placing these categories in a hierarchy based on the sequence in which they usually are mastered. The first two taxonomies were developed by committees of university experts in psychology and educational measurement. The psychomotor taxonomy was developed by a teacher of home economics. All emphasize classroom learning and provide few examples related to health care. However, because the terminology they use has become widely adopted, these books can help you find terms to express your ideas in what has become a common language for many educators.

REDMAN B K 1988 The process of patient education, 6th edn. Mosby, St Louis
> Many references on teaching include a summary of the three taxonomies just listed, but this is one of the most useful. A proposed taxonomy for perceptual learning also is described, and all systems are liberally illustrated with examples from patient education.

Even when you feel confident you know exactly what you hope to help your students learn, putting these ideas into words students and your fellow teachers can understand can be difficult. In recent decades many teachers have agreed on a common format for doing this that calls for stating objectives in terms of observable behaviors to be demonstrated by the students. To some degree this format is arbitrary and stylized so that writing objectives can seem a bit like writing Haiku or sonnets. However, the components of the format are logical and following a widely accepted system often facilitates communication. To learn to use this style, try working with either of the following self-instructional references:

MAGER R 1975 Preparing instructional objectives, 2nd edn. Fearon, Belmont, California
> Provides exercises and self-assessment tests that will help you learn to write specific objectives that describe observable indicators of learning and spell out the conditions of performance and the level of achievement needed for acceptable mastery.

TROYER D L 1971 Formulating performance objectives. In: Weigand J E (ed) Developing teacher competencies. Prentice-Hall, Englewood Cliffs, New Jersey

> Includes a pre-test, post-test and series of practice exercises that should help you achieve a useful level of skill as an objective writer in an hour or two of independent study.

Finally, remember you don't have to do all this on your own. The work of other teachers can help you both to decide what types of learning would be most valuable and to find words to explain your intent. As part of their efforts to approve (accredit) educational programs and develop licensure or registration examinations the national professional organizations in many health disciplines have published lists of the knowledge and skills new graduates should have before they enter practice. If you are planning on-the-job training for staff, job descriptions and personnel evaluation forms can be useful sources of objectives. If your responsibilities include patient and family education you will find the published literature a rich source of recommendations on what patients with frequently seen disorders need to learn. A few notable examples are:

WOLDRUM K, BOWER K, RYAN-MORRELL V, TOWSON M, ZANDER K 1985 Patient education: tools for practice. Aspen, Rockville, Maryland

> A collection of teaching plans developed by nursing staff at the New England Medical Center Hospitals in Boston. All plans are presented in a useful standard format that could easily be adopted by other disciplines, and many include samples of handouts developed to accompany teaching.

WILSON-BARNETT J (ed) 1983 Patient teaching. Recent advances in Nursing 6. Churchill Livingstone, Edinburgh

> Unlike many books which base recommendations about what patients should be taught largely on customary practices and the collective opinions of experienced staff, this reference combines practical suggestions for teaching goals and methods with a review of supporting research. It serves, therefore, not only as a good source of potential objectives, but also as a source of ideas on how the effectiveness of your efforts to help students achieve these objectives can be objectively assessed. An annotated bibliography also is included.

Commission on Education of the American Occupational Therapy Association, 1984 Guide to fieldwork education. American Occupational Therapy Association, Rockville, Maryland

> This compilation of policies, forms, guidelines and papers concerned with fieldwork education includes a guide to preparation of objectives. It is of special interest because it includes examples of enabling activities to help students achieve each goal, and because it shows differences and similarities between the objectives for students in professional and assistant level programs.

CHAPTER 3 Improving motivation & compliance

If you would like to read about practical guidelines and techniques you might use in your own teaching and at the same time learn more about the many underlying factors that can cause poor motivation and compliance the following references will serve you well.

DIMATTEO M R, DINICOLA D D 1982 Achieving patient compliance: the psychology of the medical practitioners role. Pergamon, New York

> A scholarly, humane, and practical reference. It reviews a wide range of research on topics such as: patient–practitioner relationships, rapport, models of health behavior, cultural influences, formation of behavioral intentions, and supports and barriers to behavior change. From this rich background the authors derive a series of practical guidelines for improving compliance using an approach that relies heavily on individualized negotiation of goals and methods.

REDMAN B K 1988 The process of patient education, 6th edn. Mosby, St Louis

> Reviews a wide variety of theory and research on motivation to learn and discusses its application to teaching patients. Among the topics covered are: the health belief model, provider–patient relationships, stages of psychosocial adaptation to illness, and general principles of motivation applicable to many learning situations. Practical suggestions include methods for assessing motivation as well as many for improving it.

RANKIN S H, DUFFY K L 1983 Patient education: issues, principles and guidelines. Lippincott, Philadelphia

> Describes Chatterson's adaptation of the Health Beliefs Model, and uses this as the basis for a method of mutual goal-setting and decision-making clinical teachers can use when the patient's values are in conflict with those of the health professional.

PURTILO R 1984 Health prefessional/patient interaction, 3rd edn. Saunders, Philadelphia
Written for students in the health professions, the thoughtful analysis of patient–practitioner relationships in this book can provide both students and their teachers useful insight into interpersonal sources of misunderstanding and mistrust. Discussion of such topics as incentives for getting well and advantages of staying sick provides help in understanding many patient compliance problems, while comments on the roles of students and professionals suggest ideas for helping students come to grips with the expectations held for them.

O'CONNOR A B 1986 Nursing staff development and continuing education. Little Brown, Boston
Recognizes that in teaching graduate professionals the instructor often must both interest students in learning new methods and encourage change in existing organizational practices. Motivation is discussed within the framework of theory on the process of change and review of strategies for conflict management. A humanistic approach is outlined for designing instruction and interacting with students to make new learning acceptable.

MAGER R 1968 Developing attitudes toward learning. Fearon, Palo Alto, California
An entertaining analysis of how attitudes are learned and how teachers can strengthen student interest in learning and using the information they are given. In addition to many logical comments on factors that teach students to like or dislike, seek out or avoid a subject, this book provides practical suggestions on the use of modeling and on methods for evaluating your success in stimulating students' interest.

When patients, students or staff fail to use what you have taught them, lack of motivation is usually thought to be the culprit. However, the real source of the problem may be more complex. The following two references, one theoretical and the other practical, will help you avoid approaching these problems in too simplistic a way.

BOLLES R C 1967 Theory of motivation. Harper & Row, New York
A detailed and scholarly review of the historical development of motivation theory and of research concerned with the concepts and behaviors associated with that theory. Chapters on incentive theories, secondary reinforcement and punishment discuss many topics of special relevance for clinical teaching.

MAGER R, PIPE P 1970 Analyzing performance problems. Fearon, Belmont, California
Describes a logical series of questions for step-by-step analysis of the underlying causes of poor performance. These are equally applicable to diagnosis of patient and student failure to do what we recommend. A useful flow chart leads from analysis of cause to suggested remedy.

To learn more about how to use non-authoritarian techniques for improving motivation and compliance, try several of the following:

SIMON S B, HOWE L W, KIRSCHENBAUM H 1972 Values clarification: a handbook of practical strategies for teachers and students. Hart, New York
This is the first of several books compiling exercises teachers can use to help students identify the beliefs and values they prize, examine the consequences of alternative actions, and reflect on whether their beliefs and actions are congruent. Seventy nine non-authoritarian strategies are described, each in enough detail to let you visualize it in use and decide whether it would be helpful to your own students.

STECKEL S B 1982 Patient contracting. Appleton-Century-Crofts, Norwalk, Connecticut
A detailed review of both the theoretical basis for contracting and the practical steps needed for effective design and implementation of such agreements. The emphasis is on contingency contracting, in which provision of timely and appropriate rewards plays a key role. Discussions of reinforcement theory, and techniques for decreasing unwanted behaviors and shaping new patterns of action, present many ideas that can be used either within or outside the context of a formal contract. Examples of applications include both contracts between patients and professionals, and self-change agreements staff can make with their supervisors or with themselves.

MCKAY M, DAVIS M, FANNING P 1981 Thoughts and feelings: the art of cognitive stress intervention. New Harbinger Publications, Richmond, California
Presents a fascinating array of imaginative techniques for changing undesirable patterns of habitual behavior. The methods are described in workbook format that allows you to practice using them on your own. Although the techniques were selected for their value in reducing physical and emotional reactions to stress, many have potential for changing other types of habitual behavior. Some methods, such as value clarification, visualization and problem solving are already in use by many clinical teachers. Others, such as covert assertion, stress inoculation and techniques

for combating distorted thinking, are probably less familiar. Instructions for all exercises provide fine examples of how to give clear directions to students for completing a complex learning assignment.

MILLER J (ed) 1983 Coping with chronic illness: overcoming powerlessness. F A Davis, Philadelphia
An exceptional book, notable for the clarity and humanism of its theoretical framework and for the logic and practicality of the strategies it suggests. It begins with a thoughtful review of the sources and consequences of powerlessness and of the many elements in chronic illness that may contribute to this problem. Equal attention is given to analysis of coping mechanisms patients can use and strategies by which professionals can avoid making patients feel powerless and facilitate their efforts to cope. All points are clearly illustrated with excellent case examples.

KRAMER M 1974 Reality shock: why nurses leave nursing. Mosby, St Louis
Even highly motivated staff and students may find compliance difficult when they face conflicting expectations for their behavior. This important book analyzes the frustration and anxiety new graduates in nursing experience when they try to reconcile the professional values they were taught in school with the pragmatic demands of work in a bureaucratic organization. The Anticipatory Socialization program developed by the author to help students prepare for and cope with these differences is described in terms of nursing education. However most elements of the method seem highly applicable to avoiding similar problems in many other professional fields.

CHAPTER 4 Clinical teaching methods

One good reason for exploring the literature on teaching methods is to broaden the range of techniques you feel prepared to use. If you would like to do this a good place to start is with one of the books on teaching that provides an overview of many different methods. Although in some cases the description of each technique is brief, these references will give you a useful idea of how and why the methods are used and should help you pick out new approaches to teaching you want to study in detail. Many of these books provide bibliographies that will help you locate journal articles and books that provide such detail; and many also present suggestions

on how to select methods to match particular teaching situations and purposes. Many of the references in this category have been written primarily for university lecturers, or reflect in their titles a concern with one professional discipline such as nursing or social work. Don't be discouraged by this if your work is in a different field. The techniques described in all of the following references can be easily adapted for use in a clinical setting by teachers in any health profession.

DE TORNYAY R, THOMPSON M 1983 Strategies for teaching nursing, 3rd edn. John Wiley, New York
Descriptions of a wide variety of methods are combined with practical guidelines for their use and unusually helpful explanations of rationale and related research. Methods discussed include both such familiar techniques as lectures, seminars, questions, demonstrations, and explaining through examples and models; and newer methods such as use of teaching simulations and games, self-instructional materials, and a problem-solving approach called guided design.

FOLEY R P, SMILANSKY J 1980 Teaching techniques: a handbook for health professionals. McGraw-Hill, New York
A particularly valuable feature of this book is its inclusion of checklists and rating scales you can use to evaluate your performance as you use various teaching methods. This is an especially useful reference if you would like to improve your use of already familiar techniques such as lectures, group discussion, demonstrations and questioning. It also provides many useful suggestions on teaching problem-solving skills through use of methods such as role playing, simulations and case discussions.

O'CONNOR A B 1986 Nursing staff development and continuing education. Little Brown, Boston
Brief descriptions of a broad spectrum of methods for teaching both individuals and groups are accompanied by comments on advantages and limitations, uses and practical considerations associated with each technique. Techniques discussed range from buzz groups and brainstorming to field trips, forums and case studies. Similar information is presented on an equally wide variety of teaching materials such as handouts, flip charts, bulletin boards, posters, published materials and a number of different audio-visual media. Accompanying chapters on selecting a teaching strategy and format will help you make sensible choices from this array of tools.

NARROW B 1979 Patient teaching in nursing practice: a patient and family-centered approach. John Wiley, New York
Presents brief but very useful guidelines for selecting and using techniques such as lectures, discussions, explanations, exploratory communication, live and filmed demonstrations, role playing and role modeling, and a variety of audio-visual materials.

REDMAN B K 1988 The process of patient education, 6th edn. Mosby, St Louis
This well-known reference is of special value for several reasons. Descriptions of many techniques are accompanied by samples of lesson plans and teaching materials that illustrate their use in specific patient education programs. These will help you visualize the practical process of methods such as guided imagery, contracting and mental rehearsal if you have not used them before. Other valuable features include the clear rationale for matching methods to purpose, suggestions for adapting instruction for children and for incorporating teaching into the patient's overall plan of care, and the extensive bibliographies. Best of all, however, is a major chapter on printed and non-printed teaching materials. It will help you both to locate useful published materials, and to select or produce materials your patients will find both attractive and easy to understand.

MCKEACHIE W J 1986 Teaching tips: a guidebook for the beginning teacher, 8th edn. D C Heath, Lexington, Massachusetts
It is no surprise to find this book is now in its eighth edition. The blend of practical ideas and soundly based rationale it provides has made it a classic. Although written primarily for the classroom teacher, both practicum supervisors and staff educators will find much here they can use. Lectures and group discussions receive primary attention and the reviews of research on effectiveness of these methods should help you select the method that is best matched to your needs and to use both methods skillfully. Among the many other techniques discussed are student projects and assignments, computer-assisted instruction, audio-visual techniques, one-on-one teaching and counselling, laboratory teaching and instructional games, simulations, and the case method. In each section a brief review of related research helps to explain what types of learning might benefit most from this method, and what factors influence effectiveness.

EBLE K 1977 The craft of teaching. Jossey-Bass, San Francisco
Of special interest because of its graceful style,

good humor and common sense, this book is a fine source of practical ideas on how to use such familiar techniques as the lecture effectively and also on 'survival skills' such as those needed to deal with students if they are hostile, cheat, or present other problems such as questioning the teacher's authority.

For additional references on a wide variety of both traditional and innovative teaching methods, see also the bibliography for Chapter 6. A sampling of references in which you will find quite detailed discussion of the specific methods discussed in this chapter includes:

On lectures and other methods for teaching by telling

BROWN G 1980 Lecturing and explaining. Methuen, London
Work with this book can help you make practical improvements in your performing skills both for formal lectures and unscheduled explanations. It includes several different types of useful material: guidelines and strategies for improving the clarity, audibility and relevance of what you say; instructions for practice exercises that will let you work on these skills in an orderly and enjoyable way; and rating sheets and comments by the author you can use to evaluate your strengths and weaknesses.

NEWBLE D, CANNON R 1983 A handbook for clinical teachers. MTP Press, Boston
Drawing on their work with physician educators these authors from the Advisory Centre for University Education at Australia's University of Adelaide present a wealth of useful ideas on both classroom or clinical lectures and on other presentations often expected of clinicians, such as scientific reports at conferences and poster sessions. The section on lecturing includes a list of frequently cited attributes of a good lecturer, a system for organizing content, and brief suggestions on how to combine straight lectures with discussion. A good checklist of practical points to remember when preparing for scientific presentations should be of special value for in-service and continuing education lecturers, especially if you plan to use audio-visual equipment.

On using demonstrations and coaching student practice of psychomotor skills

SINGER R 1980 Motor learning and human performance. Macmillan, New York
Includes a review of research and suggested

guidelines on such practical matters as the influence of task complexity on decisions about whether to have students practice a task as a whole or in parts, factors that influence transfer of skill from one task to another, and what type and amount of feedback is most likely to be effective at different stages of learning.

KLEINMAN M 1983 The acquisition of motor skill. Princeton Book Company, Princeton, New Jersey
A thorough review of theory and research on motor learning with especially useful chapters on transfer of training, distribution of practice, and information theory and knowledge of results.

WILLIAMS L V 1983 Teaching for the two-sided mind: a guide to right brain/left brain education. Prentice Hall, Englewood Cliffs, New Jersey
Includes a variety of thought-provoking comments and suggestions on how recent research on hemispheric specialization might be applied to teaching. The principal concern is with teaching cognitive skills; however the sections on multisensory learning and visual thinking provide an interesting framework for thinking about demonstrations and alternative systems for helping students 'get the idea' of a new motor skill.

TURNBULL G I 1986 The application of motor learning theory. In Banks M (ed) Stroke. Churchill Livingstone, Edinburgh
The other references listed here all concern teaching movement skills to students with intact neuromuscular systems. This paper is an excellent source of ideas on how your approach may need to be adapted for teaching patients with perceptual or motor deficits such as those accompanying stroke.

On structuring observations and other independent student activities

JOYCE B, WEIL M 1980 Models of teaching, 2nd edn. Prentice Hall, Englewood Cliffs, New Jersey
Among the many approaches to teaching described and analyzed in this remarkable book are several that represent very different types and amounts of teacher-initiated structuring of student activities. See, for example, the sections on non-directive teaching, the biological science inquiry approach, advance organizers and inductive thinking.

SHULMAN S, KEISLAR E R (eds) 1967 Learning by discovery: a critical appraisal. Rand McNally, Chicago
A collection of important, but primarily theoretical papers on various alternatives to expository teaching. It will help you think about the many different ways in which students can use

experience to arrive at important facts and principles without being told these by the teacher. However, this is not a particularly good source of practical guidelines for arranging and building such experiences in a clinical setting.

HENDERSON E S, NATHENSON M B (eds) 1984 Independent learning in higher education. Educational Technology Publications, Englewood Cliffs, New Jersey
This review of instructional methods used in the undergraduate and continuing education courses offered by Britain's Open University includes a section on advance organizers and related techniques for introducing students to a body of learning. Description of theory and methods for guiding the reading, experiments and projects students do on their own at home is accompanied by interesting specific examples. Many of the ideas presented could be applied to structuring student clinical assignments and to staff or student learning projects.

BARROWS H, TAMBLYN R 1980 Problem-based learning: an approach to medical education. Springer, New York
Describes a system for using carefully designed cases as the starting point and organizational framework for learning. It is an approach that not only fits well with experiences in which students are encouraged to discover key facts and principles for themselves, but also can be used to help students learn to decide for themselves what kinds of facts they need to solve patient problems.

On direct and indirect supervision of student practice

KADUSHIN A 1976 Supervision in social work. Columbia University Press, New York
A particularly helpful reference if much of the supervision you provide must be based on the student's reports of what he did and experienced rather than on your own direct observation of these events. Among the many sections of special interest are those on preparation for supervisory conferences, relationships and sources of tension between supervisors and supervisees, games supervisees may play to manipulate the level of demands made on them, practical techniques for providing support during supervision, and methods of providing educational supervision for the supervisors themselves.

YERXA E 1984 Techniques of supervision; and duties and responsibilities of fieldwork educators in the educational process. In: Commission on Education of the American Occupational Therapy Association, Guide to fieldwork education. American

Occupational Therapy Association, Rockville, Maryland

The comments on supervision in these two papers are not detailed but do present a clear view of the communication between teacher and student that can occur if supervision is treated as a constructive, two-way exchange rather than simply as an occasion when the student is told what she did wrong. A separate section of this book contains interesting examples of materials sent to students before they begin a clinical assignment to help them know what to expect. These can provide a valuable foundation for succeeding supervisory sessions by establishing a positive climate for communication and helping the students anticipate how they will be evaluated.

BENNER P 1984 From novice to expert: excellence and power in clinical nursing practice. Addison-Wesley, Nursing Division, Menlo Park, California

Experienced clinicians may have difficulty providing helpful guidance to beginners because their own work with patients often relies heavily on skilled intuitive judgment and expert interpretation of subtle cues. When the supervisor responds to things the student fails to notice, and arrives at conclusions through a process that is difficult to describe, attempts to coach performance can be frustrating for supervisor and student alike. This book can help you analyze the differences in the way the novice student or staff member sees and responds to clinical problems and the process you use as an experienced practitioner. It also presents many practical suggestions for ways in which teachers can facilitate growth from one level of competence to another through the supervision they provide.

On using questions to stimulate thinking and guide discussion

HYMAN R 1979 Strategic questioning. Prentice Hall, Englewood Cliffs, New Jersey

Suggests a system for classifying questions according to their purpose and describes a variety of systematic methods for asking questions to guide students in attempting different types of responses. Includes many examples along with useful suggestions on various practical aspects of questioning.

CUNNINGHAM R T 1971 Development of question-asking skills. In: Weigand J (ed) Developing teacher competencies. Prentice Hall, Englewood Cliffs, New Jersey

An interesting and useful self-instructional unit that includes a mixture of practical suggestions,

practice exercises and feedback. Considers such topics as how to respond to incorrect or incomplete student answers, how to involve all students in a class in discussion, and how to phrase your questions clearly.

HARGIE O, SAUNDERS C, DICKSON D 1981 Social skills in interpersonal communications. Croom Helm, London

Wording questions appropriately is only one component of effective use of discussions to foster learning. Skills in establishing an open climate for exchange of ideas and in responding constructively to student questions and answers are equally essential. This book is useful for learning the techniques needed for effective give and take in discussion and includes methods for reinforcing response, reflecting and verbal following as well as for demonstrating, explaining and providing variation.

KASULIS T P 1984 Questioning. In: Gullette M (ed) The art and craft of teaching. Harvard University Press, Cambridge, Massachusetts

Combines a realistic portrayal of the challenges involved in leading a discussion, with constructive ideas on how to phrase questions, increase student–student interaction, draw non-participants into a discussion, and encourage students to go beyond recitation of facts to suggest their own interpretation and application of ideas.

On role modeling, relationships and other techniques for influencing values

KING E C 1984 Affective education in nursing, a guide to teaching and assessment. Aspen, Rockville, Maryland

Includes both reviews of background theory on affective learning and description of selected strategies for teaching in this domain. Teaching methods discussed include values clarification exercises, group discussions, use of case studies, role playing and simulation gaming. Although most examples involve rather formal, teacher-directed activities for classroom use, many techniques can be adapted for small group use in the clinic.

BROPHY J, GOOD T 1974 Teacher–student relationships. Holt, Rinehart and Winston, New York

A scholarly review of research on this broad topic that includes a summary of the controversy surrounding Robert Rosenthal's work on the effect of teacher expectations on student achievement. It suggests methods teachers can use to think analytically about their own interaction style; and includes a description of research on the way student expectations may influence teacher behavior.

NASH R 1976 Teacher expectations and pupil learning. Routledge and Kegan Paul, London
A short but valuable book, written in refreshingly straightforward language. This provides a good introduction to ways of thinking about teacher–student interactions and the attitudes and expectations that lie behind them.

KURPIUS D 1971 Developing teacher competencies in interpersonal transactions. In: Weigand J (ed) Developing teacher competencies. Prentice Hall, Englewood Cliffs, New Jersey
Of particular value for improving your skills in both listening to and talking with individual patients, staff and students. In addition to a short review of several theories of interpersonal communication, this chapter provides a series of practice exercises you can use to build basic interpersonal skills. These include lessons on empathy, respect and concreteness, as well as a post-test and several rating scales to be used during the exercises to assess your style and skill.

OLESEN V L, WHITTAKER E W 1968 The silent dialogue. Jossey-Bass, San Francisco
This report of a landmark study of professional socialization among students in a university nursing program provides fascinating insights into the internal experience of becoming a professional. The investigators' field notes on student conversations and actions offer a revealing look at the varied ways in which students react and respond to the exhortations and expectations of those around them. Of particular interest are chapters on the art and science of studentmanship, games students and supervisors play, cycles of the inner world, and processes of becoming. Although today's students doubtless respond differently in many ways from the group studied by these authors, this book continues to provide a valuable stimulus for thinking analytically about student-supervisor roles and relationships.

Finally, regardless of the teaching methods you use most frequently you may find references on teaching aids and resources helpful. The references by O'Connor and Redman mentioned in the first part of the bibliography for this chapter will help you locate and select useful materials. Several other usually valuable guides to resources are:

HINCHCLIFF S M (ed) 1986 Teaching clinical nursing, 2nd edn. Churchill Livingstone, Edinburgh
Reviews a wide range of teaching resources and aids including a variety of audio-visual tools, flip/wall charts, programmed instruction units, models and chalkboards. Basic information on these materials are accompanied by usually sensible suggestions for their selection and use.

RANKIN S H, DUFFY K L 1983 Patient education: issues, principles and guidelines. Lippincott, Philadelphia
This is an outstanding source of information about sources of printed and audio-visual materials for use in patient education. In addition to a helpful checklist you can use to assess such materials, the book provides an extensive list of professional organizations, voluntary and non-profit groups, and commercial companies that originate and distribute patient education materials. Information provided includes patient education materials. Mailing addresses are given for each organization along with information about the focus and format of the materials it distributes. This listing is limited to organizations in the United States but should be useful to clinical teachers in most English-speaking countries.

DAVIS R M, SCHENK B 1978 Media handbook: a guide to selecting, producing and using media for patient education programs. American Hospital Association, Chicago.
An immensely practical book in which step-by-step directions for selection, production, use and evaluation of a wide variety of teaching aids are presented within an overall framework that begins with needs assessment and ends with evaluation of learning. Clear diagrams and photographs make each process easy to understand.

CHAPTER 5 Evaluation

Whether you are trying to develop your own tools for evaluating students or simply want to use an existing system more effectively, thoughtful application of the principles of sound measurement and evaluation is essential. The following general references will help you review many of the concepts and procedures that are of particular importance in this process.

THORNDIKE R L, HAGEN E 1977 Measurement and evaluation in psychology and education, 4th edn. Wiley, New York
A widely-used, easy-to-understand reference on methods for measuring learning. Of particular value for clinical teachers are the sections on

construction and use of rating scales and sources of bias in observational ratings. A helpful glossary of measurement terms and thorough discussions of validity and reliability are worth study whether you are an experienced teacher or a novice.

GRONLUND N 1988 How to construct achievement tests, 4th edn. Prentice Hall, Englewood Cliffs, New Jersey
Much of this classic text is concerned with construction of paper and pencil tests of cognitive learning. However, the introductory comments on the uses of evaluations and chapters on designing performance tests, the relationship of achievement tests to instruction, interpretation of test results and principles of validity and reliability, all have much to offer the clinical teacher. Also of special value are the clear explanations of such widely-used terms as formative and summative evaluation, and criterion-referenced and norm-referenced standards.

As you try to decide which specific aspects of performance to consider in evaluating student mastery of a need skill, validity of measurement becomes a critical issue. The following reference will help you focus your evaluations accurately.

MAGER R 1973 Measuring instructional intent, or, got a match? Fearon, Belmont, California
This light-hearted book on a serious topic describes a clear, step-by-step process for judging whether the behaviors on which you base your judgments truly match the types of learning you want to evaluate. The practice exercises and analytical flow-sheet the author provides can help you avoid many of the errors in focus that may make evaluations unfair or inaccurate.

If you would like to explore a variety of different approaches to evaluation, look at several references that present examples of many types of methods and materials suitable for use in a clinical setting. See, for example:

MORGAN M, IRBY D 1978 Evaluating competence in the health professionals. Mosby, St Louis
This informative book focuses directly on evaluation of student achievement in the clinic. It uses examples from many different health professions, and includes a valuable annotated bibliography. Samples of a variety of recording forms are accompanied by clear explanations of how these materials were developed and used. Also of special interest are the chapters on assessment of student affect, observational assessment of performance and self-assessment.

SCHNEIDER H L 1979 Evaluation of nursing competence. Little Brown, Boston
This is a particularly useful reference on methods for evaluating clinical skills through direct observation of performance. In addition to discussion and samples of varied formats for recording evaluations, such as anecdotal notes and rating scales, this book presents a detailed description of the process used to develop one specific new form, a criterion behaviors' checklist. Steps such as selection of specific behaviors to be included, testing the instrument for reliability, development of a scoring system, and use of field test results to revise the form, all are clearly explained. This provides a model process you could apply to development of your own evaluation instruments.

REILLY D E, OERMANN M H 1985 The clinical field, its use in nursing education. Appleton-Century-Crofts, Norwalk, Connecticut
Includes wise comments on such topics as the nature of clinical evaluation, the importance of fairness and a supportive climate, the use of objectives as a framework for judgments, and the value of using multiple strategies for gathering information about performance. Procedures are described in terms of student evaluation, but are equally applicable to staff. Examples include: anecdotal records, critical incident technique, rating scales and analyses of case presentations, patient care notes, and student journals. A chapter on grading suggests many useful ideas on how information about performance can be interpreted and summarized.

REDMAN B K 1988 The process of patient education, 6th edn. Mosby, St Louis
An exceptionally rich source of practical ideas on techniques for evaluating the effectiveness of patient and family instruction. Of particular value are the many sensible suggestions on how to evaluate whether patients actually follow through in using what they have learned. Among the methods discussed are patient self-reports, analysis of patient charts, oral questioning, physiologic measures, and evaluation of data from agency service reports or other documented records of patient status and use of health services.

Of special interest because they emphasize important aspects of evaluation that receive little attention in most standard texts on this subject are:

LLOYD J S (ed) 1982 Evaluation of non-cognitive skills and clinical performance. American Board of Clinical Specialties, Chicago

A fascinating collection of papers presented at a 1981 conference concerned with evaluation of such professional qualities as empathy, communication skills, manual dexterity and moral judgment, all difficult or impossible to measure using traditional written examinations. The variety of methods suggested for evaluating these qualities is unusually wide, including such techniques as peer review, medical records audit, performance checklists and interaction analyses. The examples given are proposed for use in evaluating candidates for certification in a medical specialty, but most could be used equally well in evaluating either staff or students in any discipline that involves direct patient contact.

NEUFELD V, GEOFFREY D (eds) 1985 Assessing clinical competence. Springer, New York
A valuable selection of papers written by members of the Faculty of Health Sciences at McMaster University in Toronto. Topics range from historical review of ways in which competence has been defined and measured to descriptions of such relatively new assessment techniques as medical records audits and use of patient management problem simulations. Of particular interest are chapters on direct observation, records review, global rating scales and methods for evaluating patient–practitioner relationships.

KING E C 1984 Affective education in nursing: a guide to teaching and assessment. Aspen, Rockville, Maryland
Includes a detailed chapter on construction of assessment instruments for evaluating learning of attitudes, values and beliefs. Among the methods discussed are several different types of rating scales, attitude and opinion inventories, interviews and written questions.

If you would like suggestions on how to improve your skill in giving feedback to the staff or students you supervise, see:

KADUSHIN A 1976 Supervision in social work. Columbia University Press, New York
Suggests a variety of practical techniques for giving useful feedback during individual conferences scheduled for review of staff or student performance. Sensitive comments on the nature of supportive supervision provide insight into sources of possible tension between supervisor and supervisee, and outline guidelines for avoiding confusion, anxiety and discouragement. Also included are suggestions on use of group conferences for giving feedback, and brief descriptions of alternative methods for monitoring performance when direct observation is inappropriate.

KURPIUS D 1971 Developing teacher competencies in interpersonal transactions. In: Weigand J E (ed) Developing teacher competencies. Prentice Hall, Englewood Cliffs, New Jersey
Provides practice exercises and self-evaluation scales you can use to improve your personal communication skills in specific areas such as: empathy, respect and concreteness and specificity of expression. Based on the work of humanistic psychologists, such as William Schutz, the techniques presented have broad applicability in giving non-authoritarian feedback to patients, students and staff.

To learn more about methods for helping students learn to assess themselves, and to explore the philosophy of teaching that gives this aspect of evaluation special emphasis, see:

KNOWLES M 1975 Self-directed learning. Association Press, New York
Most of this well-known author's publications on adult education include discussion of self-assessment and self-directed learning, but these topics receive particularly careful attention in this volume. This thoughtful discussion identifies the types of skills learners need in order to be self-directed, and suggests a variety of practical things teachers can do to facilitate this process.

KNOWLES M (ed) 1984 Androgogy in action. Jossey-Bass, San Francisco
A fascinating collection of papers describing adult education programs which emphasize student self-assessment and self-directed learning. Of special interest because they involve education of health professionals are chapters describing the preparation of medical students for life-long learning at Canada's McMaster University, several undergraduate programs in social work, and a hospital-based program for teaching advanced clinical skills to critical care nurses. This volume also reprints many sections of the 1978 American Nurses Association publication, Self Directed Continuing Education in Nursing. The guidelines and examples this provides could be used to good advantage by health professionals in many other fields.

GALE J 1984 Overview: self-assessment and self-remediation strategies. In: Henderson E S, Nathenson M B (eds) Independent learning in higher education. Educational Technology Publications, Englewood Cliffs, New Jersey

A scholarly analysis of how students can assess their own progress and identify activities that will help them learn. This is combined with sensible comments on why this process is important. Examples and summaries of related research are drawn primarily from work in distance learning programs such as those offered by Britain's Open University.

SMITH R M 1982 Learning how to learn: applied theory for adults. Cambridge, The Adult Education Company, New York
Provides practical guidelines clinical staff could use in designing independent study activities for their own continuing professional education. These are accompanied by interesting examples of personal learning projects, and by suggested activities and reference materials teachers can use to help students acquire self-directed learning skills. The role of self-assessment receives special attention.

HOULE C 1980 Continuing learning in the professions. Jossey-Bass, San Francisco
In addition to a valuable review of the recent efforts by many professional organizations to develop self-assessment examinations for their members, this book includes a realistic analysis of the difficulties experienced professionals often confront in evaluating their own performance. The author suggests an approach to self-monitoring that is designed to help practitioners scrutinize their own actions critically, even in areas that have become highly intuitive or habitual.

Finally, if your responsibilities include teaching patients and families, a single remarkable book will help you explore many of the different aspects of evaluation mentioned in this chapter. It is:

RANKIN S, DUFFY K 1983 Patient education: issues, principles, and guidelines. Lippincott, Philadelphia
A wide-ranging chapter on evaluation outlines an excellent list of guiding questions teachers can use as the framework for a multi-faceted evaluation of their patient teaching. It considers both the characteristics of the instructional process used and the results this process produces. The checklist is accompanied by a host of practical ideas on topics as diverse as the characteristics of good feedback, and how the results of evaluation can be documented in the patient's medical record. Useful examples are provided to show how evaluation of behavioral change related to instructional objectives can be made an integral part of overall patient care. Other sections of this fine book discuss how adult learning theory can be applied to a collaborative approach to patient

teaching, and introduce methods for evaluating the effectiveness of large scale health education programs.

CHAPTER 6 Responding to individual differences

Designing instruction tailored to the diverse needs and abilities of individual students calls first and foremost for the ability to conceive of alternatives. As teachers, many of us have difficulty moving beyond our own experience to visualize an approach that is different from the one that works best for us, or to adopt a method we never used as students. The following two superb references can help you overcome such methodological tunnel vision. Both provide solid introductions to a wide variety of teaching tools and approaches, and both make a compelling case for the value of diversity.

DE TORNYAY R, THOMPSON M 1987 Strategies for teaching nursing, 3rd edn. John Wiley, New York
A major section of this book is devoted to individualized instruction. An introductory chapter includes descriptions of seven different instruments for evaluating learning style, a review of related research emphasizing studies of nursing and allied health students, and comments on the teacher's role and on some basic techniques for responding to individual differences. Additional chapters provide a wealth of information on development and use of such tools as instructional modules, learning contracts and computer-assisted instruction.

JOYCE B, WEIL M 1980 Models of teaching, 2nd edn. Prentice-Hall, Englewood Cliffs, New Jersey
Written in the belief there is no one best way to teach, this book is of unusual interest both because it provides informative descriptions of a wide variety of different approaches to teaching, and because of the way these models are analyzed and compared. Among the 22 approaches included are methods as diverse as assertiveness training and behavior modification, role playing and inquiry method, non-directive teaching and use of advance organizers. Commonalities among models are emphasized by grouping them into four families, each representing a distinct orientation towards people and how they learn. Distinctive features and practical implications are clarified by brief scenarios describing teacher actions and student behavior when the approach is put to use.

As your familiarity with different methods grows, you may want to think about how several of them might be combined. Descriptions of the Mastery Learning approach developed by Benjamin Bloom provide a useful example of how this can be done. See, for example:

BLOCK J H (ed) 1971 Mastery learning: theory and practice. Holt, Rinehart & Winston, New York
A collection of papers on Mastery Learning, including one by Benjamin Bloom describing rationale and principal components of the method. Based on the idea that most students can achieve a high level of mastery, even of complex or difficult skills, providing they are provided with appropriate time and learning options; this approach draws on use of instructional modules, learning options, individualized feedback and self-paced study to help students with different aptitudes achieve common objectives.

For additional information on many of these specific techniques see:

McKEACHIE W J 1986 Teaching tips: a guidebook for the beginning teacher, 8th edn. D C Heath, Lexington, Massachusetts
Includes helpful sections on assignments, programmed instruction, computer uses, learning contrasts and other modular methods.

In Exercise 24 you were asked to look at some of the ways individual students may differ in choosing the process by which they find it easiest and most satisfying to learn. In recent years such differences in preferred learning style have received growing attention in educational research, and a variety of instruments now exist to measure different dimensions of these preferences. To learn more about this work and its practical implications for your clinical teaching see:

ENTWISTLE N 1981 Styles of learning and teaching. John Wiley, Chichester
This book is of special value for several reasons. It is unusually broad in scope, covering a far wider range of instruments for measuring learning style than do most references on this topic. It focuses principally on adult learners, and summarizes a wide range of interesting research. Descriptions of measurement methods are accompanied by thoughtful discussion of various conceptual models of learning style and of the many different dimensions that may be important.

Best of all, it considers the practical implications of student differences for the teacher and presents many ideas on how teachers might respond. 'Stop and think' sections throughout the book pose questions that will help you assess your own ideas on teaching and see new ways in which you might adopt a more varied approach.

HENDERSON E S 1984 Introduction: theoretical perspectives on adult education. In: Henderson E, Nathenson M (eds) Independent learning in higher education. Educational Technology Publications, Englewood Cliffs, New Jersey
Reviews a variety of different cognitive styles and learning strategies but also discusses other theoretical models of factors that influence the way individual adults learn. These include developmental models such as those of Piaget, Erikson and Kolberg, as well as motivational models such as Maslow's hierarchy of human needs.

SMITH R M 1982 Learning how to learn: applied theory for adults. Cambridge, The Adult Education Company, New York
In addition to clear summaries of many different dimensions of learning style and comments on practical implications for the teacher, this book provides a list of many of the available instruments for measuring style and gives addresses for requesting test materials and further information.

LORENS L A, ADAMS S P 1976 Entering behavior—student learning styles. In: Ford C W, Morgan M K (eds) Teaching in the health professions. Mosby, St Louis
Discusses learning styles within the general framework of learning theory and provides a good introduction to two instruments used to assess personality and learning style differences among occupational therapy students: The Canfield-Lafferty Learning Styles Inventory and the Myers-Briggs Type Indicator.

Other sections of this Handbook provide additional material on individualizing instruction. The exercises and bibliography in Chapter 2 will help you explore methods for evaluating and responding to individual differences in your students' needs, concerns and resources. The Exercise and suggested readings on Learning contracts in Chapter 3 will help you learn about this widely used method for collaborating with individual students to design learning activities that meet their needs. Finally, the references on self-assessment and self-directed learning in

Chapter 5 will help you teach your students to design personalized learning plans of their own.

CHAPTER 7 Organizing a program

As you search for a logical way to organize your instruction, a review of conceptual models in your field may be helpful. These general theories, whether they describe the nature of human development, the process of professional practice, or the meaning of health and illness, identify key elements in a complex whole and suggest how these elements are interrelated. Such a framework can be used in turn to identify integrating elements, sequencing principles and overall goals for educational activities. However, the process of selecting the most relevant model and translating it into a practical teaching plan is far from easy. Reviewing curriculum models developed by other teachers can help you see both what this involves and why it is worthwhile. A particularly helpful example that illustrates the use of a theoretical model for organizing clinical instruction is:

REILLY D E, OERMANN, M H 1985 The clinical field: its use in nursing education. Appleton-Century-Crofts, Norwalk, Connecticut
Presents a clear, thought-provoking example of a curriculum design based on a conceptual model of nursing practice. This framework provides both unifying concepts that help students integrate multidimensional instruction, and logical guidelines for sequencing activities. A detailed plan for a teaching unit on chronic pain management outlines both the progression of objectives to be achieved and the series of coordinated clinical and classroom classes through which this can be done. The emphasis on integration of practical and theoretical instruction is especially helpful. Other sections of this exceptional book compare five different models of nursing practice and comment on how such basic views of the structure of professional subject matter influence curriculum design.

Even within a brief teaching session, such as a one-day continuing education workshop or a half hour lesson for a patient, decisions about sequence can be important. The following two references will help you develop your skills in deciding where to begin and how to progress, whether you are trying to organize a program that

lasts only a short time or one spread over a period of years.

TROJCAK D 1971 Developing a competency for sequencing instruction. In: Weigand J (ed) Developing teacher competencies. Prentice-Hall, Englewood Cliffs, New Jersey
A short self-instructional program introduces five different models for looking at learning progressions and provides practice in analyzing how these would influence selection of an instructional sequence. If the models proposed by authors such as Gagné, Bloom and Taba are not familiar, this is a good way to begin learning about them.

FOLEY R, SMILANSKY J 1980 Teaching techniques: a handbook for health professionals. McGraw-Hill, New York
Provides a valuable checklist for evaluating a teaching plan which includes several items concerned with progression of activities and adequacy of opportunities for repeated student practice. To help you learn to use the checklist, detailed outlines are presented for two different plans for a course on basic interviewing skills. Each is followed by a critique by the authors with which you can compare your own assessment.

Integration of learning is especially difficult when important components of instruction are planned by people who have little direct contact with one another. This is often the case when professionals receive their continuing education through lectures and workshops sponsored by a variety of different organizations, when patients are taught by staff from several different departments, and when fieldwork supervision is provided by clinicians who are not formally employed as faculty by the university at which students receive the didactic part of their professional education. The following references provide useful examples of methods clinical teachers in a variety of settings have designed to deal with this problem.

O'CONNOR A B 1986 Nursing staff development and continuing education. Little Brown, Boston
Suggests use of an overall conceptual framework or curriculum composed of organizing themes to provide cohesiveness, logical progression, and need repetition in staff development and continuing education programming. This is illustrated by a sample skills–responsibility matrix that could be used to organize a variety of program offerings into a connected program for nursing leadership development.

BECK S J, LE GRYS V A 1988 Clinical laboratory education. Appleton and Lange, Norwalk, Connecticut
Describes the Learning Vector Model, a logical system for progressing and integrating student responsibilities during several different stages of professional education. Both in academic coursework and clinical experiences students move through the stages of exposure, acquisition and integration as instruction progresses from early teacher-directed activities towards an end goal of student-initiated independent practice. Practical guidelines for using the model appear easy to apply in many professional fields.

SHEAFOR B W, JENKINS L E 1982 Quality field instruction in social work. Longman, New York
Includes several chapters concerned with the place of fieldwork experience in the overall professional curriculum. These suggest how efforts to make clinical application of abstract theory learned in the classroom can help students integrate otherwise fragmented knowledge. Various patterns for structuring fieldwork are described, along with valuable ideas on use of a developmental model of learning to sequence activities.

PIERCE P, EICHENWALD S 1978 Integrating didactic and clinical education—low patient contact; and Scanlan G L 1978 Integrating didactic and clinical education—high patient contact. Both in: Ford C (ed) 1978 Clinical education for the allied health professions. Mosby, St Louis
Two short but useful chapters outlining models for curriculum integration, the first particularly applicable in fields such as medical records administration or medical laboratory technology in which staff are concerned primarily with provision of diagnostic or information support services, the second most relevant for fields such as dietetics or occupational therapy in which staff have frequent direct contact with individual patients.

ALEXANDER M 1983 Learning to nurse: integrating theory and practice. Churchill Livingstone, Edinburgh
Describes experimental use of a method of coordinated classroom instruction and supervised clinical work designed to help student nurses integrate theory and practice. Of special interest are the convincing examples of student comments on the insights and encouragement they gained from this sensibly planned direct experience with the clinical phenomena they were studying in the classroom.

PRAVIKOFF D S 1983 Continuity and transition in patient education: cardiac rehabilitation in acute and outpatient settings. In: Rankin S H, Duffy K L, Patient education: Issues, principles and guidelines. Lippincott, Philadelphia
Discusses the careful instructional planning needed to meet the changing needs of patients as they progress from acute illness to convalescence and to coordinate the teaching of the many different professionals this may involve. A practical example of how such a patient education curriculum can be designed is provided through description of the cardiac rehabilitation program offered by a nurse, dietitian, physical therapist and others at one hospital.

Finally, several important references you should know, because of the great influence they have had on thinking about the education of health professionals, are:

BENNER P 1984 From novice to expert: excellence and power in clinical nursing practice. Addison-Wesley, Menlo Park, California
A revealing analysis of the nature of professional skill acquisition in which a generic model of this process developed by Dreyfus and Dreyfus is applied to nursing. The book provides both general descriptions and a wealth of specific examples of the ways in which clinical judgment changes as the professional progresses from the rule-governed, rigid, fragmented performance of the novice towards the fluid, holistic, intuitive practice of the expert. In addition to practical suggestions on how students and staff can be helped to progress through each of the five levels described, the author provides a number of interesting ideas on the nature of integrated learning and its importance in setting patient care priorities and providing holistic care.

BARROWS H, TAMBLYN R 1980 Problem based learning: an approach to medical education. Springer, New York
Describes the system of carefully designed problems and patient simulations used as the organizing framework for instruction by the Faculty of Health Sciences at McMaster University in Toronto. Although this is used as a substitute and complement for hands-on work with real patients, the model of clinical reasoning and ideas on how this reasoning can be taught have obvious applicability to such traditional clinical teaching techniques as case conferences and guidance of student work on individual patient care plans.

BARROWS H 1985 How to design a problem-based curriculum for the pre-clinical years. Springer, New York
Extends the earlier book and provides many practical suggestions on methods for using both real and simulated patients to help students

integrate theoretical and practical learning of clinical skills such as interviewing, examining and selecting treatment. Although the primary emphasis is on pre-clinical instruction, this book also stresses the need for early patient contact and proposes how clinical tutors can make that experience more valuable through coaching that uses a socratic method rather than one that simply presents information.

APPENDIX
LOCATING HELPFUL REFERENCES IN
PROFESSIONAL JOURNALS

As the introduction to this Handbook explained, the suggestions for further reading at the end of each chapter are limited to books in English, most of them issued by major publishers during the late 1970s and 1980s. This selection was based on the author's belief that such references would provide the most varied and readily accessible sources of additional reading for most teaching clinicians. This is, however, only a starting point. Journals provide an equally rich and more current source of information on many important educational topics. Here, then, are a few suggestions on how you can extend your reading into the journal literature.

BIBLIOGRAPHIES IN BOOKS

A logical place to begin looking for useful journal articles is in the bibliographies provided by authors of the suggested books. Some of these are annotated, others are not, but all cite many journal articles of particular value. Although most papers in these lists are several years old by the time the book is published, these references have been carefully selected to include key papers drawn from the journal literature over a period of many years. They will help you both to locate specific papers on topics of special interest and to identify journals you may want to consult on a regular basis in the future because of the types of articles they publish.

NATIONAL LIBRARY OF MEDICINE MATERIALS

The most comprehensive source of information about the international biomedical journal literature is:
 Index Medicus, published monthly by the National Library of Medicine, 8600 Rockville Pike, Bethesda Maryland 20894. Provides information on nearly 25 000 articles each month from over 3400 journals published in many different countries and languages. The journals indexed include many that regularly publish papers on patient education or the education of health professionals. You will find the Index in

the reference collection of most medical school and teaching hospital libraries throughout the world and in the reference collections of Universities and higher education institutes with nursing or allied health programs.

If you are near a library that has a computer link with the National Library of Medicine, and want to locate a thorough list of articles on a selected topic you may want to arrange for a computerized literature search through:
 MEDLINE, the computerized listing of journal references maintained by the National Library of Medicine as part of its Medical Literature Analysis and Retrieval System (MEDLARS). This listing includes over five million articles published in the international biomedical literature since MEDLINE was established in 1966. It accesses, in addition to Index Medicus, the International Nursing Index. Over 270 nursing journals from all over the world are indexed, as are nursing articles in the 3000 allied health and biomedical journals covered by this database.

If a computerized search is not practical for you, consider one of the 'Recurring Bibliographies' published by the National Library of Medicine on selected topics of wide interest. These include:

- the *Recurring Bibliography on Education in the Allied Health Professions* — published annually and available from the Medical Communications Division, School of Allied Medical Professions, the Ohio State University, 1583 Perry Street, Columbus, Ohio 43210
- the *International Nursing Index* — a quarterly, published by the American Journal of Nursing Company, 555 West 57th Street, New York, N Y 10019
- the *Bibliography on Medical Education* published monthly and printed as a regular section of the Journal of Medical Education (see description of that journal later in this Appendix).

You can learn more about the services of the National Library of Medicine by talking to the reference librarian at most large health science libraries, National Library of Medicine materials and services also are available to readers in the UK through Health

Board/Authority libraries, the library of the King's Fund Institute, 126 Albert Street, London NW1 7NS, and in Scotland from the Scottish Health Service Centre Library

CUMULATIVE INDEX TO NURSING AND ALLIED HEALTH LITERATURE (CINAHL)

An additional source of information on the current journal literature is this Index, published as 5 bi-monthly issues and an annual cumulative volume. It is available through the Glendale Adventist Medical Center, PO Box 871, Glendale, California 91209-0871. Most English Language journals in nursing are covered as well as primary journals in 13 allied health fields. While many of these also are indexed in the National Library of Medicine materials, some valuable sources are listed only in CINAHL.

SELECTED JOURNALS ON EDUCATION IN THE HEALTH PROFESSIONS

Most journals published for clinicians in the health professions include occasional articles on various aspects of patient teaching or on the education of staff and students in the field. The many fine journals in the general field of education also provide an important source of references for clinical teachers. The bibliographies and literature search systems mentioned earlier will help you find your way to helpful material in these sources. However, you also should consider looking regularly at one or more of the specialized journals published primarily for health professionals who teach. Because those fields are especially large and well established, many of these journals focus on education in nursing or in medical schools. However, you will find many ideas you can use whether your own teaching is in those disciplines or in a different profession. Several particularly useful journals are:

● On patient, family and community education:
   Patient Education and Counseling
   6 issues annually, published by Elsevier Scientific Publishers Ireland Ltd, PO Box 85, Limerick, Ireland. An interdisciplinary, international journal that includes papers on applied research as well as commentaries on administrative issues involved in providing patient education and counseling.

Journal of Nutrition Education
Published bimonthly by George F. Stickley Company, 210 W. Washington Square, Philadelphia, Pennsylvania 19106 for the Society for Nutrition Education.
   Includes reports of projects and research related to nutrition education, along with short commentaries

on issues and programs of current interest. Of special value are the book reviews, abstracts and summaries of information on a wide variety of nutrition education materials.

Health Education Research: Theory and Practice
Published quarterly by IRL Press Limited, PO Box 1, Enysham, Oxford, OX8 1JJ, UK.
   Deals with a broad range of issues in health education and promotion. Focuses on communication as a central process and aims for practical results. A forum for researchers and practicing health educators.

Health Education Journal
Published quarterly by the Health Education Authority, 78 New Oxford Street, London WC1A 1AH.
   Each issue contains approximately 10 papers on research, education and evaluation of studies.

● On continuing education and staff development for health professionals:

Journal of Continuing Education in Nursing
Published bimonthly by Slack Inc., Thorofare New Jersey, 08086.
   Includes a wide variety of original articles reporting on research, innovative programs, trends, and issues in continuing education and staff development. A regular feature of this journal is a short section on Teaching Tips by Signe Cooper that provides many practical ideas on specific teaching methods.

Journal of Nursing Staff Development
Published quarterly by Lippincott, Philadelphia, Pennsylvania 19105.
   Articles emphasize practical information and discussion of trends and issues related to in-service educational programs for hospital staff.

● On education of students in the health professions:

Journal of Medical Education
Published monthly by the Association of American Medical Colleges, One DuPont Circle, N.W., Washington DC 21202.
   Major articles report on research in medical education and describe innovative programs in the field. Brief communications share information on new methods and report preliminary findings from trial projects. Book reviews and the monthly listing of journal articles related to medical education prepared by the National Library of Medicine's MEDLARS program will help you monitor new additions to the literature.

Journal of Nursing Education
Published 9 times yearly by Slack Inc., Thorofare, New Jersey 08086.
   Research on a wide range of topics related to nursing education is reported in major articles, while

'briefs' share ideas about new teaching techniques and views on curriculum and other issues of interest to faculty. Although many papers focus on classroom education or overall program planning, most issues include at least one paper directly concerned with a topic of interest to clinical instructors.

Medical Education

Published bimonthly for the Association for the Study of Medical Education by Blackwell Scientific Publications Ltd, Edinburgh EH3 6AJ, Scotland.

Includes papers on both research and innovative projects in medical education undergraduate, postgraduate and continuing education programs both within the United Kingdom and overseas.

Nurse Educator

Published bimonthly by J. B. Lippincott, Hagerstown, Maryland 21740.

Intended primarily for academic faculty and administrators of university programs, but often includes papers on topics of equal concern to instructors who supervise students in the clinic.

Nurse Education Today

Published bimonthly by Churchill Livingstone, Edinburgh EH1 3AF, Scotland.

Includes research reports, review articles, and accounts of new developments in education at both the basic and post-basic levels. Informative book reviews provide help in locating new references.

Both editorial board and contributors are drawn from nursing education in the United Kingdom and a number of other British Commonwealth countries and Scandinavia.

Nursing Times

Published weekly by Macmillan Magazines Limited, 4 Little Essex Street, London WC2R 3LF.

This is the largest selling nursing journal in the UK and regularly includes a Nurse Education Supplement.

Journal of Advanced Nursing

Published bi-monthly from 1976–88 and monthly since January 1989 by Blackwell Scientific Publications, Osney Mead, Oxford OX2 0EL.

Contains scholarly contributions on all aspects of nursing care and nursing education, management and research.

Physical Therapy Education

Published twice yearly by the Section for Education of the American Physical Therapy Association.

This very new journal is currently distributed primarily to members of the Education Section, but clearly has much to offer a much wider audience. Inquiries concerning subscriptions may be sent to the business manager, Scott Minor, 128 Tahoma Road, Lexington, Kentucky 40503.

Papers include research reports and descriptions of innovative progams, many of them directly concerned with clinical education. The book reviews cover both recent publications in general education and those in a variety of health professions.

INDEX